MRI of the Head and Neck

Second Edition

The LWW MRI Teaching File Series

SERIES EDITORS

Robert B. Lufkin

William G. Bradley, Jr.

Michael Brant-Zawadzki

MRI of the Brain I

William G. Bradley, Jr., Michael Brant-Zawadzki, and Jane Cambray-Forker

MRI of the Brain II

Michael Brant-Zawadzki, Jane Cambray-Forker, and William G. Bradley, Jr.

MRI of the Spine

Jeffrey S. Ross

MRI of the Head and Neck

Robert B. Lufkin, Alexandra Borges, Kim N. Nguyen, and Yoshimi Anzai

MRI of the Musculoskeletal System

Karence K. Chan and Mini Pathria

Pediatric MRI

Rosalind B. Dietrich

The LWW MRI Teaching File Series

MRI of the Head and Neck

Second Edition

Editors

ROBERT B. LUFKIN, M.D.

Professor of Radiological Science
Chief of Head and Neck Radiology
Department of Radiology
UCLA School of Medicine
Los Angeles, California

KIM N. NGUYEN, M.D.

Assistant Professor
Department of Radiology
UCLA School of Medicine
Los Angeles, California

ALEXANDRA BORGES, M.D.

Department of Radiology
Instituto Portuges de Oncologia
Lisbon, Portugal

YOSHIMI ANZAI, M.D.

Assistant Professor
Department of Radiology
University of Michigan
Ann Arbor, Michigan

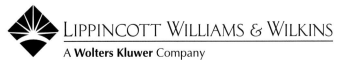

LIPPINCOTT WILLIAMS & WILKINS

A **Wolters Kluwer** Company

Philadelphia · Baltimore · New York · London
Buenos Aires · Hong Kong · Sydney · Tokyo

Acquisitions Editor: Joyce-Rachel John
Developmental Editor: Ellen DiFrancesco
Production Editor: Maria Tortora
Manufacturing Manager: Tim Reynolds
Cover Designer: Jeane Norton
Compositor: Maryland Composition
Printer: Maple Press

© 2001 by LIPPINCOTT WILLIAMS & WILKINS
530 Walnut Street
Philadelphia, PA 19106 USA
LWW.com

Printed in the USA

Library of Congress Cataloging-in-Publication Data

MRI of the head and neck / editor, Robert B. Lufkin.—2nd ed.
    p. ; cm.—(The LWW MRI teaching file series)
    Includes bibliographical references and index.
    ISBN 0-7817-2572-0 (alk. paper)
    1. Head—Magnetic resonance imaging—Case studies.   2. Neck—Magnetic resonance imaging—Case studies.   I. Lufkin, Robert B.   II. Series.
    [DNLM: 1. Head—pathology—Case Report.   2. Magnetic Resonance Imaging—Case Report.   3. Neck—pathology—Case Report. WE 705 M939 2000]
RC936 .M75 2000
617.5'107548—dc21

                                                                            00-055879

10 9 8 7 6 5 4 3 2 1

DEDICATION

To all of our families

To my grandmother Inês
Alexandra Borges

To my husband Satoshi and our new arrival Erika,
who make my life worthwhile
Yoshimi Anzai

PREFACE

MRI has assumed a key role in the diagnosis and treatment of diseases of the head and neck. Most authorities agree that skull base and nasopharyngeal lesions are best seen on MR images. The parapharyngeal spaces, oral cavity, and larynx can also be shown to advantage with the availability of axial, sagittal, and coronal images. We have selected 100 cases that cover the major problems encountered in MR examinations of the head and neck. The purpose is to present clinical cases in a format that allows the reader to develop their skills of observation as well as interpretation. Each case presented is first visualized on the left-hand page. The reader is encouraged to try to identify the pathology from these images before reading the discussion on the right-hand page that details the MR findings as well as the clinical problem. Suggested readings are also provided to the interested observer.

It is our sincere hope that anyone who wishes to become more knowledgeable in the area of head and neck, and especially in MRI, can use this book to enhance their clinical knowledge, as well as their MR interpretive skills.

We would also like to thank the staff at Lippincott William & Wilkins, including Andrea Kim, Joyce-Rachel John, and Ellen DiFrancesco, for all their help and encouragement with this project.

Robert B. Lufkin, M.D.
Alexandra Borges, M.D.
Kim N. Nguyen, M.D.
Yoshimi Anzai, M.D.

MRI of the Head and Neck

Second Edition

CASE 1

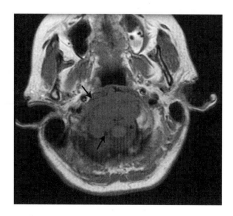

FIGURE 1.1A

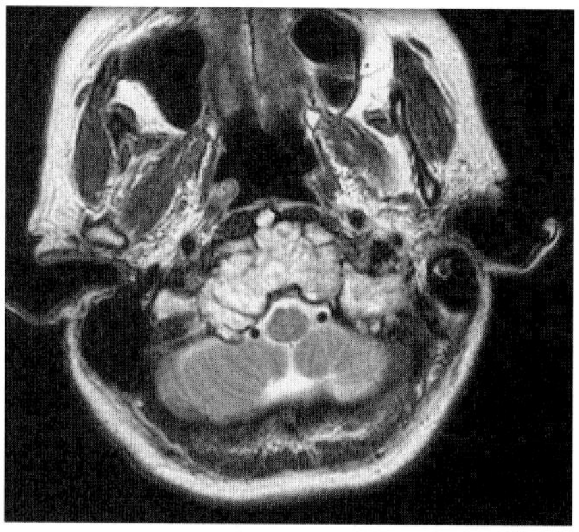

FIGURE 1.1B

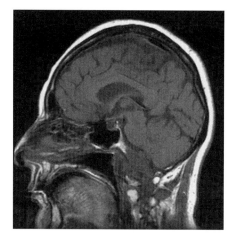

FIGURE 1.1C

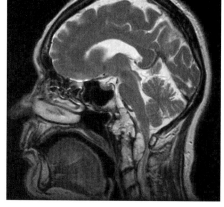

FIGURE 1.1D

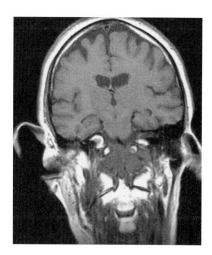

FIGURE 1.1E

CLINICAL HISTORY

A 69-year-old woman presented with headaches and a right twelfth cranial nerve palsy.

FINDINGS

The axial T1-weighted image (T1WI) shows a large soft tissue mass replacing the clivus, basiocciput, and atlas (Fig. 1.1A). The mass is grossly midline in position showing a larger right lateral component invading the ipsilateral hypoglossal canal. It is high signal on T2-weighted image (T2WI) (Fig. 1.1B). The sagittal T1WI and T2WI show the inferior extent of the mass along the ventral aspect of the epidural space to the level of the mid-C2 vertebral body (Fig. 1.1C–D). The ventral subarachnoid space is effaced and the cervical spinal cord is compressed.

The coronal T1WI shows similar findings (Fig. 1.1E).

DIAGNOSIS

Clival chordoma, chondroid variant, middle, lower level.

DISCUSSION

Chordomas are relatively rare tumors of the skull base, accounting for 1% of all intracranial tumors and 4% of all primary brain tumors. Fifty percent of chordomas arise in the sacrococcygeal region. Other common locations include the clivus and the spine, which comprise 35% and 15% of all chordomas, respectively. Intracranially, the most common locations are the basisphenoid and basiocciput (near the sphenooccipital synchondrosis) and the parasellar region. Rarely, chordomas may arise in the nasopharynx or within the paranasal sinuses. The incidence of chordomas varies according to their location. Clival chordomas can occur at any age but show a peak incidence in the third and fourth decades. Sacrococcygeal chordomas tend to present later in the 40- to 60-year-old age group. There is a male predominance.

The presenting symptoms depend on tumor location, extent, and relationship between the tumor and vital skull base structures. Most patients with clival chordomas present with headaches and ophthalmoplegia, usually resulting from impingement upon the sixth nerve in Dorello's canal. More extensive lateral extension into the cavernous sinus results in cavernous sinus syndrome with deficits of cranial nerves III, IV, V1, and V2. Posterior and inferior extension into the jugular foramen presents with palsy of cranial nerves IX, X, and XI. Involvement of the hypoglossal canal results in twelfth nerve palsy. Destruction of the petrous apex and involvement of the cerebellar pontine angle (CPA) cistern may cause deficits of the seventh and eighth cranial nerves. Anterior growth into the sella may lead to compression of the pituitary gland and hypopituitarism. Symptoms of brainstem compression and increased intracranial pressure signal advanced disease. Destruction of the occipital condyles and extension of tumor through the foramen magnum into the upper cervical spinal canal may result in neck pain and tetraparesis.

Chordomas are histologically benign, locally invasive, slow-growing neoplasms that originate from the primitive notochord. Because the embryonic notochord terminates at the sphenoid bone, immediately below the sella turcica, the midline basisphenoid is the most common location for this tumor. However, because of the intimate relationships of the notochord with several neuroectodermal, mesodermal, and endodermal derivatives, giving rise to the diencephalon, primitive pharynx, Rathke's pouch, and facial bones, other "ectopic" locations including intradural, nasopharyngeal, sellar, and sinonasal regions are possible. Notochordal remnants in the nasopharynx are believed to be responsible for the development of Tornwaldt cysts. Uncommonly, these notochordal remnants may give rise to a chordoma in these locations.

Histologically, the tumor is composed of translucent cells that are rich in mucin and glycogen and that contain a large intracytoplasmic vacuole. These physaliferous cells are usually arranged in cords or nests, separated by thick fibrous septa. Macroscopically, the tumor forms a white, soft, multilobulated mass surrounded by a pseudocapsule, composed by compressed adjacent tissues. Gelatinous mucoid fluid, necrosis, hemorrhage, and sequestered bony fragments are not infrequent and contribute to the heterogeneous imaging appearance of these neoplasms. Most chordomas are cytologically benign. The high frequency of recurrence is explained by microscopic extensions of tumor into the adjacent tissues, which, together with a difficult surgical access, make complete resection problematic. Highly malignant forms of chordoma are also seen; these contain undifferentiated areas that may be confused with fibrosarcoma. Metastasis is seen in 7% to 14% of cases, primarily to lymph nodes, lungs, and bone.

Chondroid chordoma, a variant rich in chondroid material, is a controversial pathologic entity that is believed by some to represent a low-grade chondrosarcoma. Immuno-histochemical stains are helpful in differentiating chordomas from chondrosarcomas, which may have the same appearance on imaging studies. Whereas chordomas are positive for epithelial markers such as cytokeratin and epithelial membrane antigens, chondrosarcomas are negative for epithelial antibodies but positive for mesenchymal markers such as vimentin and protein S-100. Confusion between chordomas and epithelial metastasis to the skull base may occur with immunohistochemical analysis.

Radiologic evaluation of skull base tumors should include CT scanning, MRI study, or both to determine the full bony and soft tissue extent. Depending on their location within the clivus, chordomas are classified as upper, middle, or lower clival chordomas. Upper clival chordomas occur rostral to the trigeminal nerve in the region of the dorsum sella. Middle clival chordomas occur between the origin of the fifth and ninth cranial nerves. Lower chordomas are below the origin of the glossopharyngeal nerve. Chordomas vary in size from 1 to 10 cm but most are in the 2- to 5-cm range.

Typically, these tumors arise in the midline clivus near the sphenooccipital synchondrosis. They may extend laterally into the cavernous sinus and petrous apex, anteriorly into the sphenoid sinus, superiorly into the sellar and suprasellar regions, inferiorly into the foramen magnum, or posteriorly into the jugular foramen and prepontine cistern.

MRI signal characteristics are variable depending on the presence of tumoral calcification, hemorrhage, or cystic degeneration. Usually, these tumors tend to be isointense to hypointense on T1WI and heterogeneously hyperintense on T2WI. A lobulated, honeycomb appearance after gadolinium administration has been described as a characteristic feature of chordomas. MRI is the optimal modality to detect small intraclival tumors that manifest as an area of T1W hypointensity within the high signal intensity of fat. However, care should be taken to avoid mistaking areas of hematopoietic bone marrow for a clival tumor. To avoid this confusion, one should carefully look for loss of signal void of the cortical margin of the clivus or bony erosion on CT. MRI is also the modality of choice to evaluate the relationship of the tumor to the structures of the cavernous sinus, jugular foramen, and posterior fossa and is particularly useful for identifying the presence of compression or encasement of the basilar or cavernous carotid arteries.

Despite the continuous advances in skull base surgery, most chordomas cannot be completely resected because of their tendency toward microscopic invasion and because of the proximity of important structures such as cranial nerves and major intracranial arteries. Even so, surgical excision should be attempted because radiation therapy is usually not effective in decreasing the bulk of tumor. However, radiation using high-dose proton beam therapy can be successful in the treatment of residual tumor. The choice of the best therapeutic approach is based on many factors including tumor location, clinical condition of the patient, and history of previous surgery or radiation therapy. Radiologic follow-up is mandatory because of the high rate of recurrence of these neoplasms.

SUGGESTED READINGS

Casals MM, Hunter SB, Olson JJ, et al. Metastatic follicular thyroid carcinoma masquerading as a chordoma. *Thyroid* 1995;5:217–221.

Doucet V, Peretti-Viton P, Figarella-Branger D, et al. MRI of intracranial chordomas. Extent of tumour and contrast enhancement: criteria for differential diagnosis. *Neuroradiology* 1997;39:571–576.

Kaufman BA, Francel PC, Roberts RL, et al. Chondroid chordoma of the lateral skull base. *Pediatr Neurosurg* 1995:23:159–165.

Keel SB, Bhan AK, Liebsch NJ, et al. Chondromyxoid fibroma of the skull base: a tumor which may be confused with chordoma and chondrosarcoma. A report of three cases and review of the literature. *Am J Surg Pathol* 1997;21:577–582.

Maira G, Pallini R, Anile C, et al. Surgical treatment of clival chordomas: the transsphenoidal approach revisited. *J Neurosurg* 1996;85:784–792.

Tashiro T, Fukuda T, Inoue Y, et al. Intradural chordoma: case report and review of the literature. *Neuroradiology* 1994;36:313–315.

Weber AL, Brown EW, Hug EB, et al. Cartilaginous tumors and chordomas of the cranial base. *Otolaryngol Clin North Am* 1995;28:453–471.

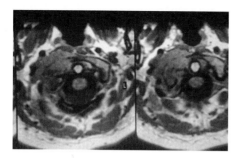

FIGURE 2.1A

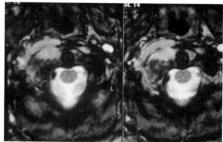

FIGURE 2.1B

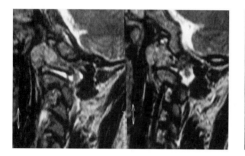

FIGURE 2.1C

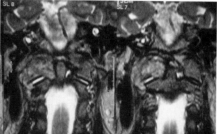

FIGURE 2.1D

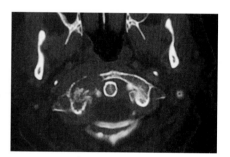

FIGURE 2.1E

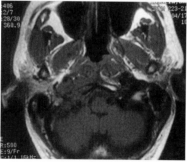

FIGURE 2.2A

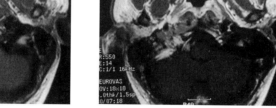

FIGURE 2.2B

CLINICAL HISTORY

A 54-year-old woman with a history of retroperitoneal leiomyosarcoma presents with suboccipital neck pain after a motor vehicle accident.

FINDINGS

Axial T1-weighted image (T1WI) and T2-weighted image (T2WI), and sagittal and coronal T2WI (Fig. 2.1A–D) through the skull base and craniovertebral junction show a soft tissue mass replacing the bone marrow of the right lateral mass and right aspect of the anterior arch of the clivus, destroying cortical bone. This is best seen on the axial CT section (Fig. 2.1E). The mass extends anteriorly into the perivertebral space, displaces the right longus colli muscle, the nasopharyngeal carotid space, and the right vertebral artery. There is no evidence of epidural extension. The dens, occipital condyle, hypoglossal canal, and jugular foramen are free of tumor.

Axial precontrast and postcontrast T1WI through the skull base (another patient) show an enhancing soft tissue mass centered at the right jugular foramen, replacing the bone marrow of the clivus and extending along the right hypoglossal canal into the right aspect of the premedullary cistern and compressing the right vertebral artery (Fig. 2.2).

DIAGNOSIS

Craniovertebral junction metastasis.

DISCUSSION

Metastasis should always be considered in the differential diagnosis of a craniovertebral destructive mass. Most cases occur in the setting of a known malignancy but, in a minority of cases, a craniovertebral metastasis is the first sign of an occult malignancy. Neoplasms that are more likely to metastasize to this region in adulthood include prostate, breast, lung, renal cell, and thyroid cancers and melanoma. Except for prostate and some breast metastases that are predominantly osteoblastic, the metastases are lytic lesions with a soft tissue component. Thyroid and renal cell cancer metastases are usually highly vascular and may be expansile and bubbly in appearance.

Besides hematogenous spread, craniovertebral lesions may occur via direct extension or perineural spread, most commonly from nasopharyngeal squamous cell carcinoma. Primary bone tumors including chondrosarcomas, osteosarcomas, plasmacytomas, lymphomas, eosinophilic granulomas, and giant cell tumors should also be considered in the differential diagnosis. Chordomas are central skull base lesions with a typical midline location centered at the sphenooccipital synchondrosis. When involving the jugular foramen, metastases may mimic glomus jugulare or glomus vagale (Fig. 2.2).

Metastases to the skull base and craniovertebral junction have been classified by Posner and Greenberg into five different categories according to the location and skull base structures involved, resulting in different clinical syndromes. Most patients present with headaches and cranial nerve deficits. When the lesion is centered in the posterior skull base, the most commonly involved structures are the jugular foramen and the hypoglossal canal.

CT and MRI should be used in combination to characterize both the bony destructive changes and the soft tissue components of the lesion. CT may add useful information, increasing the diagnostic specificity. The presence of chondroid calcifications or bony matrix, the pattern of bony destruction, and the presence of skull base neural foraminal enlargement are clues to the correct diagnosis. MRI is very sensitive to bone marrow replacement and early perineural spread of tumor before neural foraminal enlargement can be appreciated. Whereas bone marrow replacement is best seen on the precontrast T1WI, the ideal sequence to detect perineural spread is postgadolinium fat-suppressed T1WI. Most metastases are isointense to hypointense on T1WI and hyperintense on T2WI, and show contrast enhancement.

Specific features such as a "salt and pepper" appearance in highly vascular metastases and high T1W signal in melanoma and mucinous tumors may be seen.

Metastatic disease to the skull base and craniovertebral junction is managed according to the location, cell type of the primary tumor, and presence of metastases in other locations. Surgery, radiation therapy, and chemotherapy are all possible options and need to be suited to the individual case.

SUGGESTED READINGS

Lindsberg M. Bilateral sphenoid wing metastases of prostate cancer presenting with extensive brain edema. *Eur J Neurol* 1999;6:363–366.
Manolidis S. Malignant glomus tumors. *Laryngoscope* 1999;109:30–34.
Ng SH. MRI in recurrent nasopharyngeal carcinoma. *Neuroradiology* 1999;41:855–862.
Sakata K. Prognostic factors of nasopharynx tumors investigated by MR imaging and the value of MR imaging in the newly published TNM staging. *Int J Radiat Oncol Biol Phys* 1999;15;43:273–278.
Shames D. Neuromuscular oropharyngeal dysphagia secondary to bone metastases. *Conn Med* 1998;62:451–453.

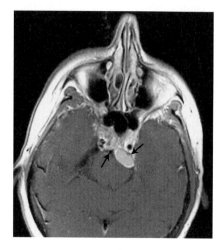

FIGURE 3.1A

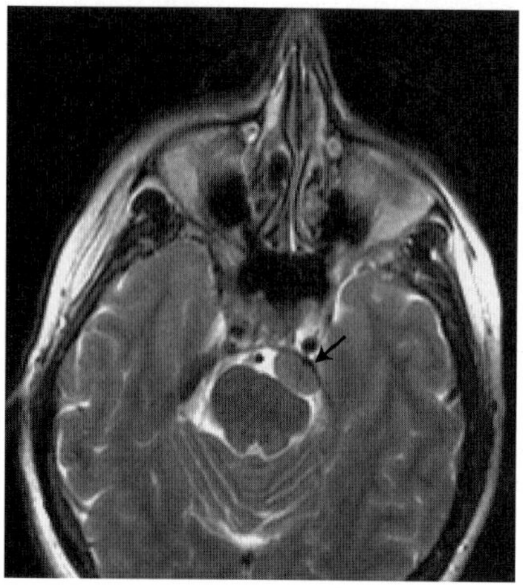

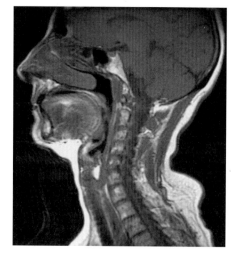

FIGURE 3.1C

FIGURE 3.1B

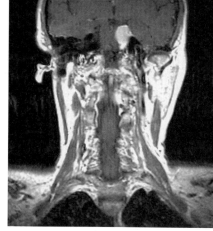

FIGURE 3.1D

CLINICAL HISTORY

A 59-year-old woman presented with a 2-year history of pain and paresthesia involving the left side of her face.

FINDINGS

Axial T1-weighted image (T1WI) MRI of the skull base shows a discrete, ovoid, extraaxial mass located in the left prepontine cistern (Fig. 3.1A). The lesion is isointense to gray matter on both T1WI and T2-weighted image (T2WI) (Fig. 3.1B). On the postcontrast images, linear enhancement is seen extending along the posterior aspect of the petrous ridge and posterosuperiorly along the tentorium (dural tail) (Fig. 3.1C). The lesion indents the left cerebral peduncle but there is a definite cleavage plane between these structures. The coronal and sagittal images show similar findings (Fig. 3.1D).

DIAGNOSIS

Petroclival meningioma (tentorial type).

DISCUSSION

Meningiomas constitute approximately 15% to 20% of intracranial neoplasms. However, tumors arising from the skull base are much less common. The most frequent sites of origin are the sphenoid ridge, cribriform plate, parasellar region, clivus, cerebellopontine angle, tentorium, and cavernous sinus. These tumors are more frequent in female patients and the peak age at presentation is in the sixth decade.

Patients with petroclival meningiomas usually present with cranial nerve palsies or, uncommonly, with signs of increased intracranial pressure when the tumors are large enough to cause obstructive hydrocephalus. Cerebellar signs may also be present. The cranial nerves involved depend on the exact tumor location. Deafness, vertigo, and tinnitus are common presenting symptoms when the tumor impinges upon the cisternal segment of the seventh and eighth nerve complex or grows along the internal auditory canal (IAC). Involvement of the trigeminal nerve in its cisternal segment or in the Meckel's cave results in trigeminal neuralgia or facial hypesthesia. Diplopia is also a frequent presenting symptom that results from compression of the sixth nerve. This may occur in its cavernous segment or in its epidural course passing through Dorello's canal. The other cranial nerves coursing in the cavernous sinus (III and IV) may also be involved. Headaches, imbalance, and papilledema can be the presenting symptoms in patients with large tumors. Other focal neurologic findings may result from brainstem or cerebellar compression. When small and separate from cranial nerves, petroclival meningiomas can be completely asymptomatic, discovered incidentally on imaging performed for other reasons.

Meningiomas are benign tumors that arise from meningothelial cells. Petroclival meningiomas originate from the meningeal folds surrounding the junction of the occipital bone, petrous apex, and sphenoid bone.

CT and MRI are the techniques of choice for imaging skull base meningiomas. MRI is particularly helpful in defining the exact location of the tumor and pattern of spread, factors critical in selecting the best surgical approach. On MRI, meningiomas are seen as well-defined globular or plaquelike masses that are isointense to gray matter on both T1WI and T2WI. Intense homogeneous enhancement is usually seen, unless calcification is present. Because of the multiplanar capability and high soft tissue contrast of MRI, it is possible to determine the site of tumor attachment and relation to the adjacent cranial nerves. Petroclival meningiomas may extend inferiorly into the jugular foramen and along the tentorium, laterally into the IAC or anteriorly into the cavernous sinus, Meckel's cave, and medial cranial fossa. The signal characteristics of meningiomas allow ready differentiation from petroclival cystic lesions.

The treatment for skull base meningiomas is surgical resection. Radiation therapy is usually considered for incomplete resections and recurrences. More recently, stereotactic radiosurgery has been used in the primary treatment of skull base meningiomas when surgical resection is expected to cause unacceptable neurologic deficits or to treat postsurgical macroscopic disease. This modality appears to allow control of further growth without severe morbidity and is a promising technique in the management of these benign, slow-growing tumors.

SUGGESTED READINGS

Couldwell WT, Fukushima T, Giannotta SL, et al. Petroclival meningiomas: surgical experience in 109 cases. *J Neurosurg* 1996;84:20–28.

Fazi S, Barthelemy M. Petroclival meningioma mimicking the presentation of a transient ischemic attack. *Acta Neurol Scand* 1994;89:75–76.

Kawase T, Shiobara R, Ohira T, et al. Developmental patterns and characteristic symptoms of petroclival meningiomas. *Neurol Med Chir* 1996;36:1–6.

Nicolato A, Ferraresi P, Foroni R, et al. Gamma knife radiosurgery in skull base meningiomas. Preliminary experience with 50 cases. *Stereotact Funct Neurosurg* 1996;66(Suppl 1):112–120.

Pomeranz S, Umansky F, Elidan J, et al. Giant cranial base tumours. *Acta Neurochir* 1994;129:121–126.

Sekhar LN, Wright DC, Richardson R, et al. Petroclival and foramen magnum meningiomas: surgical approaches and pitfalls. *J Neurooncol* 1996;29:249–259.

Tatagiba M, Samii M, Matthies C, et al. Management of petroclival meningiomas: a critical analysis of surgical treatment. *Acta Neurochir Suppl* 1996;65:92–94.

Thomas NW, King TT. Meningiomas of the cerebellopontine angle. A report of 41 cases. *Br J Neurosurg* 1996;10:59–68.

Zentner J, Meyer B, Vieweg U, et al. Petroclival meningiomas: is radical resection always the best option? *J Neurol Neurosurg Psychiatry* 1997;62:341–345.

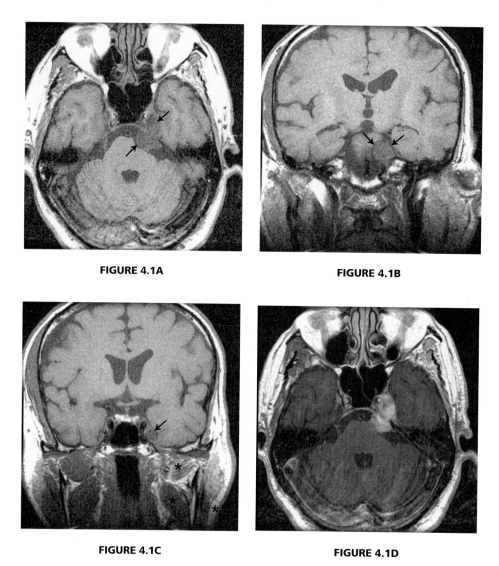

FIGURE 4.1A

FIGURE 4.1B

FIGURE 4.1C

FIGURE 4.1D

CLINICAL HISTORY

A 42-year-old woman presents with progressive left-sided facial pain and paresthesia.

FINDINGS

Axial and coronal T1-weighted MRI shows a dumbbell-shaped lesion involving the left prepontine cistern and left Meckel's cave following the course of the trigeminal nerve. This mass expands Meckel's cave and produces mass effect upon the left ventral aspect of the pons (Fig. 4.1A–C). There is atrophy and fatty infiltration of the left masticator muscles, consistent with denervation atrophy. The axial postcontrast images show enhancement of the mass with no evidence of extracranial invasion (Fig. 4.1D).

DIAGNOSIS

Trigeminal nerve schwannoma.

DISCUSSION

Schwannomas are benign nerve sheath tumors arising from cranial, spinal or peripheral nerves. They occur exclusively in sensory or mixed nerves. Intracranial schwannomas make up 8% of all intracranial tumors. Among these, 95% originate from cranial nerve VIII. Trigeminal schwannoma, although in a distant second place, is the nerve most commonly involved in the central skull base. It occurs with equal frequency in men and women, with a peak incidence in the fourth decade. Trigeminal schwannomas may occur in isolation or in association with neurofibromatosis.

Most patients present with pain, paresthesia, and numbness, usually along the course of the first or second divisions of the trigeminal nerve. The association of trigeminal schwannoma with trigeminal neuralgia is controversial. Some authors associate this neuralgic pain with involvement of the trigeminal root, whereas others relate it to involvement of the gasserian ganglion. Headaches and symptoms of compression of adjacent cranial nerves are not uncommon. Diplopia, facial weakness, and sensorineural hearing loss are among the most frequent manifestations, resulting from compression of the cavernous segment of cranial nerve VI and cisternal segments of cranial nerves VII and VIII by large trigeminal tumors. Extension of tumor along the third division of the fifth nerve may result in trismus or weakness of the masticator muscles. Large tumors in the posterior fossa may cause cerebellar and pyramidal symptoms. Extension along the V1 division may present with exophthalmos and papilledema.

Trigeminal schwannomas are benign encapsulated tumors that originate from the nerve sheath. They are composed of two different types of tissue designated as Antoni A and Antoni B (see Case 87). These tumors grow slowly, do not tend to recur, and rarely show malignant transformation. Malignant trigeminal schwannomas "de novo" are also rare, with only a few cases having been described in the literature; they are more common in the setting of neurofibromatosis (plexiform neurofibroma). These malignant tumors are characterized by increased cellularity and nuclear pleomorphism, and may be confused with sarcomas, specifically with fibrosarcoma. Most malignant trigeminal schwannomas in the head and neck are localized in the retromaxillary or pterygomandibular region.

Cross-sectional imaging allows precise depiction of tumor location and extent and has largely improved the outcome of surgical treatment. Imaging is also helpful in establishing the diagnosis and in the follow-up of these patients. CT and MRI are used complementarily to assess both bony changes and soft tissue extent, respectively.

MRI is the best imaging modality to assess the extent of these tumors. Gadolinium-enhanced MRI may depict small tumors that would otherwise be missed. Trigeminal schwannomas tend to be isointense to brain on T1-weighted images and hyperintense on T2-weighted images, and enhance after contrast administration. Fluid–fluid levels resulting from hemorrhage or layering of debris or fluids with different protein composition have been reported in these lesions.

MRI better delineates the relationship of the tumor to adjacent structures, particularly with the brainstem, petrous apex, seventh and eighth nerve complex, cavernous sinus, and intracranial segments of the internal carotid artery. Replacement of the fat signal adjacent to the skull base foramina and pterygomaxillary fissure is a useful sign of tumor extension into these foramina and is better depicted with noncontrast T1-weighted images. Cross-sectional studies for patients with trigeminal nerve symptoms should include all segments of the nerve, including the posterior fossa, skull base, orbits, and infratemporal fossa. Atrophy and fatty infiltration of the muscles of mastication may be seen, indicating denervation atrophy. This imaging finding should prompt a search for trigeminal nerve pathology.

The treatment for trigeminal schwannomas is surgical excision. The surgical approach is dictated by the location and extent of the tumor. The best management of malignant schwannomas appears to be surgery followed by radiation therapy.

SUGGESTED READINGS

Catalano P, Fang-Hui E, Som PM. Fluid-fluid levels in benign neurogenic tumors. *AJNR Am J Neuroradiol* 1997;18:385–387.

Charabi S, Mantoni M, Tos M, et al. Cystic vestibular schwannomas: neuroimaging and growth rate. *J Laryngol Otol* 1994;108:375–379.

Krishnamurthy S, Holmes B, Powers SK. Schwannomas limited to the infratemporal fossa: report of two cases. *J Neurooncol* 1998;36:269–277.

Mautner VF, Lindenau M, Baser ME, et al. The neuroimaging and clinical spectrum of neurofibromatosis 2. *Neurosurgery* 1996;38:880–886.

Samii M, Migliori MM, Tatagiba M, et al. Surgical treatment of trigeminal schwannomas. *J Neurosurg* 1995;82:711–718.

Tegos S, Georgouli G, Gogos C, et al. Primary malignant schwannoma involving simultaneously the right gasserian ganglion and the distal part of the right mandibular nerve. Case report. *J Neurosurg Sci* 1997;41:293–297.

Turgut M, Palaoglu S, Akpinar G, et al. Giant schwannoma of the trigeminal nerve misdiagnosed as maxillary sinusitis. A case report. *South Afr J Surg* 1997;35:131–133.

Yamashiro S, Nagahiro S, Mimata C, et al. Malignant trigeminal schwannoma associated with xeroderma pigmentosum—case report. *Neurol Med Chir* 1994;34:817–820.

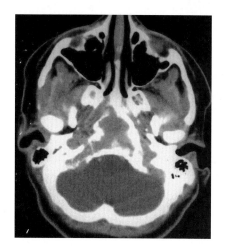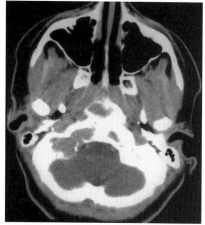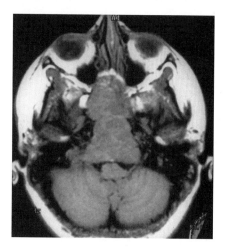

FIGURE 5.1

FIGURE 5.2

FIGURE 5.3

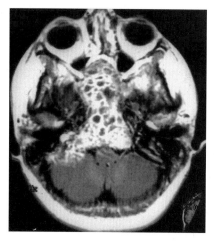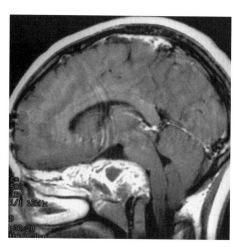

FIGURE 5.4

FIGURE 5.5

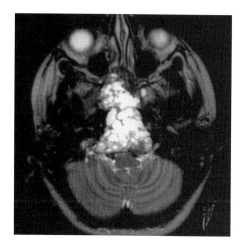

FIGURE 5.6

CLINICAL HISTORY

A 13-year-old girl presents with headache, nausea, right eye pain, and photophobia. No cranial nerve symptoms were present.

FINDINGS

CT scan shows a multiloculated, well-defined osteolytic lesion involving the clivus and occipital condyle, extending to the sphenoid sinus (Fig. 5.1). The bone margin is expansile rather than destructive (Fig. 5.2). MR shows a complex cystic lesion diffusely involving the entire clivus and occipital bones (Fig. 5.3–5). The clivus and sphenoid sinuses are enlarged, associated with mild compression of the ventral aspect of the brain stem. T2-weighted images show multiple small cystic lesions surrounded by a low signal rim, suggestive of presence of hemorrhage(Fig. 5.6). Fluid–fluid level is also seen.

DIAGNOSIS

Aneurysmal bone cyst (ABC).

DISCUSSION

Aneurysmal bone cyst (ABC) is an expansile lesion containing thin-walled, blood-filled cystic cavities. This is considered nonneoplastic in nature. Trauma is thought to be important in pathogenesis in some ABCs. The local alteration of blood flow may play a role in development of ABC, which usually occurs in the first, second and third decades of life and which frequently involves long tubular bone and spine. Within the long bones, ABC arises from the metaphysis. The posterior elements are the most common sites for spinal ABC. A patient with skull ABC may present with moderate to severe headache or sometimes focal neurologic symptoms. ABC often appears as an expansile osteolytic lesion with fluid–fluid level on CT. This fluid–fluid level, however, can be seen in other skull lesions, such as giant cell tumor and chondrosarcoma. MR shows low signal on T1- and high signal on T2-weighted images, surrounded by low T2 signal rim. The lesion may contain a single cystic cavity or more frequently a meshwork of multiple cysts.

Differential diagnosis should include giant cell tumor, chordoma, chondrosarcoma, chondroblastoma, hemangioendothelioma, hemorrhagic metastasis, and telangiectatic osteosarcoma. Mucocele of the sphenoid sinus may have a similar radiographic appearance.

SUGGESTED READINGS

Resnick D. Bone and joint imaging. In Resnick D, ed. *Tumor and tumor like disease.* Philadelphia: WB Saunders, 1989;1107–1182.

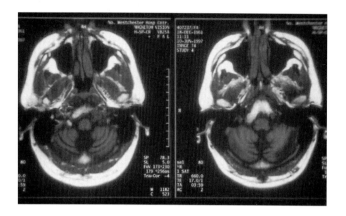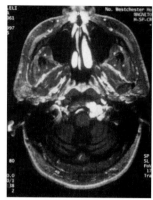

FIGURE 6.1A

FIGURE 6.1B

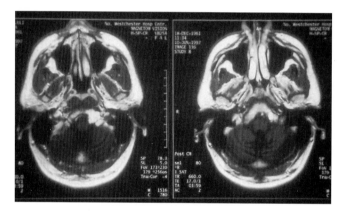

FIGURE 6.1C

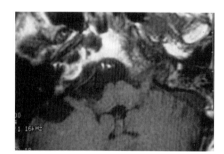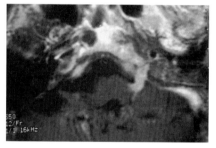

FIGURE 6.2A

FIGURE 6.2B

CLINICAL HISTORY

A 36-year-old man presents with fasciculations and atrophy of the left hemitongue.

FINDINGS

Axial T1-weighted, T2-weighted, and gadolinium-enhanced T1-weighted images through the posterior fossa (Fig. 6.1A–C) show a grossly pear-shaped mass with intraaxial and extraaxial components centered at the left hypoglossal canal. The intracranial component obliterates the lateral aspect of the premedullary cistern and surrounds the left vertebral artery (seen better on the axial precontrast T1-weighted images). The lesion extends along the hypoglossal canal into the nasopharyngeal carotid space behind the left longus colli muscle. There is remodeling of the left lateral aspect of the clivus and enlargement of the hypoglossal canal when compared with the contralateral side.

The mass is lobulated in contour, is isointense to brain on T1-weighted, is hyperintense on T2-weighted images, and enhances vividly and homogeneously. Axial precontrast and postcontrast T1-weighted images (Fig. 6.2A and 2B [another patient]) show enlargement and linear, diffuse enhancement along the cisternal and hypoglossal canal segments of the left cranial nerve XII (retrograde perineural spread of recurrent nasopharyngeal carcinoma).

DIAGNOSIS

Hypoglossal nerve schwannoma.

DISCUSSION

Hypoglossal schwannomas are rare and, in most cases, are associated with neurofibromatosis type II. They are benign slow-growing tumors presenting late, usually with compressive symptoms of adjacent structures. The hypoglossal nerve is the single lower cranial nerve that exits the intracranial compartment in a separate foramen. After exiting the brainstem at the preollivary sulcus, the hypoglossal nerve traverses the premedullary cistern as several separate rootlets in close proximity to the vertebral artery, which join together to enter the hypoglossal canal. From there, the nerve curves caudally within the high carotid space joining the remainder of the lower cranial nerves in their inferior course.

Isolated hypoglossal symptoms point to the lesion site within the cisternal or intracanalicular segments of the hypoglossal nerve. Larger tumors compress adjacent structures, mainly the other lower cranial nerves at the jugular foramen or carotid space, medulla, and, when the tumor extends inferiorly through foramen magnum, the cervical spinal cord.

On clinical examination, there is tongue deviation to the side of the lesion on protusion, tongue atrophy, and fasciculations. Patients may also complain of dysarthria and suboccipital headaches.

MR is the best imaging modality to evaluate tumor extent and may be helpful in the differential diagnosis with other situations that may present with lower cranial nerve neuropathy. Besides neural tumors of the lower four cranial nerves, other considerations include clival meningiomas, epidermoids, glomus vagale and glomus jugulare, clival tumors such as eccentric chordomas and chondrosarcomas, and skull base metastasis.

Similarly to other nerve sheath tumors, hypoglossal schwannomas are isointense to brain on T1-weighted and hyperintense on T2-weighted images, and they tend to enhance vividly as most tumors are highly vascularized. A heterogeneous MR appearance may be seen in large tumors that undergo cystic degeneration or hemorrhage.

Contrast-enhanced MR may be the only way to detect small tumors manifesting as a small focal area of nodular enhancement along the course of the nerve. Perineural spread of malignancies along cranial nerve XII is not uncommon, and when this situation is suspected, care should be taken to include all the course of the nerve, from the brainstem to the hyoid bone, within the imaging study as this type of spread may be discontinuous, showing "skip lesions." CT demonstrates remodeling and erosion of the hypoglossal canal and, if the tumor is large enough, erosion of the jugular foramen and clivus.

Management of hypoglossal schwannomas is surgical, usually through a suboccipital craniotomy.

SUGGESTED READINGS

Bung G. Dumb-bell hypoglossal neurinoma with intra- and extracranial paravertebral expansion. *Acta Neurochir (Wien)* 1998;140:1209–1210.

Chong VF. Hypoglossal nerve palsy in nasopharyngeal carcinoma. *Eur Radiol* 1998;8:939–945.

Kachhara R. Large dumbbell neurinoma of hypoglossal nerve: case report. *Br J Neurosurg* 1999;13:338–340.

Karpati RL. Synchronous schwannomas of the hypoglossal nerve and cervical sympathetic chain. *AJR Am J Roentgenol* 1998;171:1505–1507.

Omura S. Oral manifestations and differential diagnosis of isolated hypoglossal nerve palsy: report of two cases. *Oral Surg Oral Med Oral Pathol Oral Radiol Endod* 1997;84:635–640.

Sato M. Hypoglossal neurinoma extending intra- and extracranially: case report. *Surg Neurol* 1996;45:172–175.

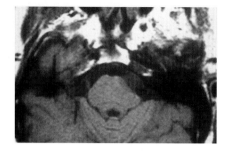
FIGURE 7.1A

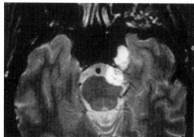
FIGURE 7.1B

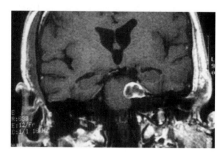
FIGURE 7.1C

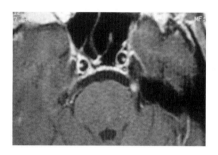
FIGURE 7.2A

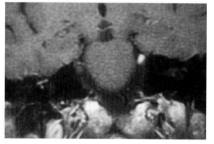
FIGURE 7.2B

CLINICAL HISTORY

A 73-year-old man presents with left-sided facial pain and paresthesias.

FINDINGS

Axial T1-weighted and T2-weighted and gadolinium-enhanced coronal T1-weighted images through the skull base (Fig. 7.1A–C) show a heterogeneous mass centered in the left prepontine cistern and Meckel's cave along the course of the left trigeminal nerve. The mass is partially cystic, hypointense on T1-weighted images, and hyperintense on T2-weighted images, and it shows irregular marginal enhance-ment. There is mass effect upon the pontomesencephalic junction. The foramen ovale is normal in appearance without evidence of extracranial spread of tumor.

Axial (Fig. 7.2A) and coronal (Fig. 7.2B) gadolinium-enhanced T1-weighted MR images (another patient) show a 5-mm focus of nodular enhancement in the cisternal segment of the left trigeminal nerve.

DIAGNOSIS

Trigeminal schwannoma.

DISCUSSION

Schwannomas account for 5% to 10% of all intracranial tumors. Among these, 95% originate in cranial nerve VIII, followed at distance by trigeminal tumors. Trigeminal schwannomas may present at any age, but a peak incidence is reported in the fourth decade. When associated with other central nervous system tumors (schwannomas or meningiomas), trigeminal schwannomas are part of the spectrum of neurofibromatosis type II. These tumors may occur anywhere along the course of cranial nerve V, including the intracranial and extracranial segments, and they have different clinical presentations according to their location.

The most common location for trigeminal schwannomas is the middle cranial fossa (type I tumors), accounting for 50% of all tumors, usually arising from the gasserian ganglion. The tumor begins to enlarge Meckel's cave and then extends anterior and laterally into the middle cranial fossa or cavernous sinus. Tumors in this location tend to present with facial pain and facial paresthesias in one or more fifth nerve distributions. Involvement of the cavernous sinus results in other cranial nerve deficits (cavernous sinus syndrome). Tumors in the posterior fossa (type II) arise in the prepontine cistern from the retrogasserian trigeminal roots and account for 20% of all tumors. Symptoms result from compression of adjacent structures, usually the brainstem and structures of the cerebellopontine angle. Twenty-five percent of tumors have both posterior and middle cranial fossa components (type III) and assume a bi-lobed, dumbbell shape because of tumor constriction at the porus trigeminus, such as in this case. A combination of clinical findings results. Finally, schwannomas may arise from trigeminal nerve branches and manifest as an extracranial mass. Usually, these tumors extend intracranially through their natural foramina (superior orbital fissure, foramen rotundum, and foramen ovale).

In most cases, tumors are relatively large at the time of diagnosis and may be difficult to resect completely, leading to recurrences. Not uncommonly, large tumors show important cystic and mucinous degeneration, mimicking other cystic lesions.

In the setting of neurofibromatosis type II (except for plexiform neurofibromas), malignant trigeminal schwannomas are rare and usually peripheral in location.

Imaging, particularly MR, provides excellent delineation of tumor boundaries and extent, and is useful in the diagnosis, treatment planning, and follow-up. CT may be used complementarily to access any associated bony changes such as bone remodeling, erosion, or foraminal enlargement. Small tumors, less than 1 cm in size, may only be detected on gadolinium-enhanced MR images (Fig. 7.2A, B). Larger tumors are hypointense to isointense to gray matter on T1-weighted images and hyperintense on T2-weighted images, and they enhance after intravenous contrast. When cystic degeneration or hemorrhage occurs, the tumor becomes more heterogeneous and may show fluid–fluid levels. Important tumor relationships for treatment planning include the following: brainstem, petrous apex, cerebellopontine angle structures (seventh and eighth cranial nerves complex), cavernous sinus, and intracranial internal carotid artery. Extension along trigeminal branches is best depicted on precontrast T1-weighted images (by replacement of fat signal within or adjacent to skull base neural foramina), and in fat-suppressed gadolinium-enhanced T1-weighted images (by abnormal foraminal enhancement). Denervation atrophy of the muscles of mastication should prompt a search for a trigeminal nerve lesion and imaging studies need to include all the course of the nerve from the brainstem to the mandible.

The major differential diagnoses include petroclival or cavernous sinus meningiomas, other cranial nerve schwannomas (usually vestibular or facial schwannomas), and epidermoid cysts. Hyperostosis and the presence of a dural tail favors the diagnosis of meningioma. Vestibular schwannomas are usually more lateral in location, centered at the porus acusticus, and tend to enlarge the internal auditory canal. Facial nerve schwannomas, similarly to trigeminal schwannomas, may extend into the middle cranial fossa and assume a dumbbell appearance. Extension of the lesion into the geniculate ganglion, located in the anterior and superior aspect of the petrous bone, favors the facial nerve as the nerve of origin. Other possible causes of nodular enhancement of the trigeminal nerve include perineural spread of tumor, metastases, or inflammatory conditions.

The presence of skip-enhancing nodules along the course of the nerve is typical for perineural spread of tumor in that schwannomas grow by direct extension along the nerve sheath and are rarely multicentric. Hematogenous metastases from breast and lung carcinomas and from melanoma are also a possibility in this setting.

Trigeminal schwannomas are managed surgically. Radiation surgery may be an option for inoperable or recurrent tumors.

SUGGESTED READINGS

Catalano P, Fang-Huui E, Som PM. Fluid-fluid levels in benign neurogenic tumors. *Am J Neuroradiol* 1997;18:385–387.

Dominguez J. Surgical findings in idiopathic trigeminal neuropathy mimicking a trigeminal neurinoma. *Acta Neurochir (Wien)* 1999;141:269–272.

Huang CF. Stereotactic radiosurgery for trigeminal schwannomas. *Neurosurgery* 1999;45:11–16.

Krishnamurthy S, Holmes B, Powers SK. Schwannomas limited to the infratemporal fossa: report of two cases. *J Neurooncol* 1998;36:269–277.

Majoie CB. Primary nerve-sheath tumours of the trigeminal nerve: clinical and MRI findings. *Neuroradiology* 1999;41:100–108.

Osterhus DR. Trigeminal schwannoma. *Am J Otol* 1999;20:551–552.

Yoshida K. Trigeminal neurinomas extending into multiple fossae: surgical methods and review of the literature. *J Neurosurg* 1999;91:202–211.

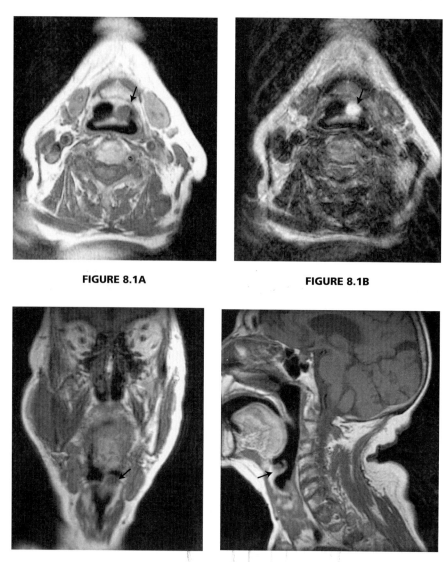

FIGURE 8.1A   FIGURE 8.1B

FIGURE 8.1C   FIGURE 8.1D

CLINICAL HISTORY

A 55-year-old male presents with chronic cough.

FINDINGS

Axial T1-weighted images of the neck show a 1.5-cm well-defined, hypointense, round lesion in the left vallecula, posteroinferior to the tongue base (Fig. 8.1A). The lesion is hyperintense on T2-weighted images (Fig. 8.1B). No invasion of surrounding structures is noted. The coronal and sagittal views confirm these findings (Fig. 8.1C,D).

DIAGNOSIS

Vallecular cyst.

DISCUSSION

Vallecular cysts are retention cysts that arise as a result of obstruction of mucous glands. Although anatomically the vallecula is not part of the larynx, pathologically it may be considered as part of the larynx. In the pediatric age group, supraglottic cysts at the tongue base and vallecula comprise the majority of laryngeal cysts. Vallecular cysts usually present in infancy with equal male-to-female ratios and are uncommon in adulthood. Most infants present with feeding difficulty, failure to thrive, stridor, or respiratory distress. Early diagnosis and a high index of suspicion are required because these lesions may cause life-threatening airway obstruction. Adults may present with difficulty swallowing, fullness in the throat, referred ear pain, or stridor when the lesion is large and impinges on the laryngeal vestibule.

Histologically, vallecular cysts are true epithelial-lined cysts. Association with laryngomalacia, probably secondary to extrinsic compression by the cyst, has been described in which a redundant epiglottis prolapses into the laryngeal vestibule during inspiration. Removal of the cyst usually leads to resolution.

Lateral projection radiographs of the soft tissues of the neck are useful in children presenting with stridor. Supraglottic cysts manifest as an abnormal soft tissue density, posterior to the tongue base, obliterating the vallecula and displacing the epiglottis posteriorly.

On CT or MRI, a vallecular cyst manifests as a fluid-containing, nonenhancing lesion centered in the vallecula, posterior to the base of the tongue. The degree of airway obstruction and displacement of the epiglottis should be assessed and the surgeon alerted to the need for a tracheostomy before any procedure is attempted.

Coronal or sagittal MRI may better delineate these lesions and show their full extent. It also assists in differentiating vallecular cysts from other cystic lesions such as thyroglossal duct cyst (TGDC), tongue base cyst, and laryngocele. TGDC tends to be more midline and have a more anterior location between the strap muscles and the hyoid bone or thyroid ala. Internal laryngoceles grow superiorly in the paraglottic space and tend to displace the vallecula superiorly. In children, ectopic thyroid tissue should be excluded and the presence of a thyroid gland in normal anatomic position confirmed by radionuclide thyroid scan before surgery.

Vallecular cysts may be managed by marsupialization and laser ablation. Endoscopic aspiration has a high rate of recurrence.

SUGGESTED READINGS

Guitierrez JP, Berkowitz RG, Robertson CF. Vallecular cysts in newborns and young infants. *Pediatr Pulmonol* 1999;27:282–285.

Kamble VA, Lilly RB, Gross JB. Unanticipated difficult intubation as a result of an asymptomatic valecular cyst. *Anesthesiology* 1999;91:872–873.

Oluwole M. Congenital vallecular cyst: a cause of failure to thrive. *Br J Clin Pract* 1996;50:170.

Wang CR, Lim KE. Vallecular cysts: report of two cases. *Pediatr Radiol* 1995;25(Suppl 1):S218–S219.

Wong KS, Li HY, Huang TS. Vallecular cyst synchronous with laryngomalacia: presentation of two cases. *Otolaryngol Head Neck Surg* 1995;113:621–624.

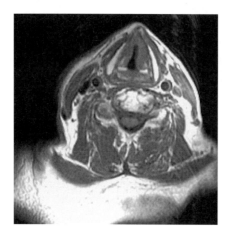

FIGURE 9.1A

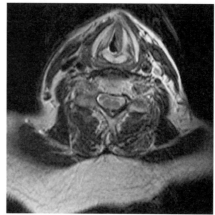

FIGURE 9.1B

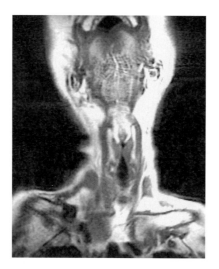

FIGURE 9.1C

CLINICAL HISTORY

A 50-year-old male becomes hoarse over the past 3 months.

FINDINGS

T1-weighted axial sections through the true vocal cords show a fullness in the left true cord musculature extending to the anterior commissure and widening that structure (Fig. 9.1A). On T2-weighted images, there is increased signal intensity (Fig. 9.1B).

The coronal T1-weighted MRI (Fig. 9.1C) shows no evidence of extension beyond the true cords. The paralaryngeal space is clear.

DIAGNOSIS

Squamous cell carcinoma of the vocal cord.

DISCUSSION

Because glottic cancers involve the vocal cords, they present very early with hoarseness. Nodal spread is rare in the case of early lesions because there is an absence of lymphatics along the free margin of the vocal cords. Advanced lesions with a fixed cord, however, have a higher incidence of lymphatic involvement. Because these tumors are readily accessible, most are diagnosed and managed by clinical examination using laryngoscopy and biopsy. The primary role of CT and MRI, therefore, is to define the extent of disease for appropriate management.

Glottic tumors (arising from the true cords) are the most common laryngeal cancers, typically affecting males in their fifth to seventh decades. Of malignancies of the larynx, 90% are squamous cell carcinomas and these tumors are usually well differentiated. Glottic cancers are slow-growing lesions that tend to metastasize late as a result of the limited lymphatic drainage of the vocal cords. Initially, most patients complain of intermittent hoarseness that progressively worsens. These tumors have been linked to smoking and radiation exposure.

Seventy-five percent of these tumors involve the anterior half of the true vocal cord as in this patient. Early glottic lesions (staged at T1) have an excellent prognosis; the 5-year survival rate approaches 95% with surgery or radiation therapy. Cross-sectional imaging of these lesions may show thickening of the true cords or they may be normal. If the clinician has a clear view and can confirm that the lesion is an early T1 tumor, MRI is not necessary. With more advanced tumors and because the signals from tumor and muscle differ, the distinction between exophytic lesions and lesions infiltrating the true cord musculature is well demonstrated. True cord tumors spread to involve the mucosa over the arytenoids or at the anterior commissure.

Therefore, even though they are the most common laryngeal cancers, they are not the most common laryngeal cancer in radiology departments because imaging studies add little to the diagnostic workup in most cases. The very early true cord tumor can be readily evaluated on indirect clinical examination and does not generally require an imaging study. The more advanced lesions that show extension to the anterior commissure regions above or below the vocal cord are a different matter. They require imaging techniques to show deep infiltration and full extent of the tumor.

Glottic cancers are staged according to the following system:

T1—Limited to vocal cords
T2—Extends to supraglottic or subglottic, or with impaired cord mobility
T3—Limited to larynx with cord fixation
T4—Invades thyroid cartilage or extralaryngeal spread

Cord fixation may be the result of several mechanisms. Tumor may infiltrate the intrinsic laryngeal musculature and fix the cord to the thyroid cartilage. Bulky tumor may limit cord mobility by mass effect or may involve the cricoarytenoid joint. Scans may show an arytenoid cartilage in the median or paramedian position. MR can show how the spread to the deep tissue planes and cartilage invasion lead to fixation. Only rarely is fixation due to causes other than tumor, such as rheumatoid arthritis.

Mucosal spread to the false cord may not be appreciated with MRI; however, extension across the ventricle to the false cord via the paralaryngeal space decreases the fatty high signal deep to the cord. Coronal sections are particularly useful because bulky lesions occasionally bulge upward, distorting the false cords rather than invading them. This may be difficult to appreciate on axial images.

T1 and T2 lesions may be treated with surgery or radiation. Spread to the false cord and significant subglottic spread may necessitate a vertical hemilaryngectomy. Further extension may fix the vocal cord to produce a T3 lesion, which may worsen the prognosis and make selection of the appropriate therapy potentially more difficult. Advanced lesions with cartilage invasion or extensive infraglottic spread generally require total laryngectomy.

SUGGESTED READINGS

Katsounakis J, Remy H, Vuong T, et al. Impact of magnetic resonance imaging and computed tomography on the staging of laryngeal cancer. *Eur Arch Otorhinolaryngol* 1995;252:206–208.

Mukherji SK, Castillo M, Huda W, et al. Comparison of dynamic and spiral CT for imaging the glottic larynx. *J Comput Assist Tomogr* 1995;19:899–904.

Teresi LM, Lufkin RB, Hanafee WN. Magnetic resonance imaging of the larynx. *Radiol Clin North Am* 1989;27:393–406.

Weinstein GS, Laccourreye O, Brasnu D, et al. The role of computed tomography and magnetic resonance imaging in planning for conservation laryngeal surgery. *Neuroimaging Clin North Am* 1996;6:497–504.

CASE 10

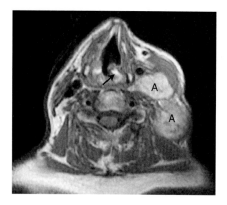 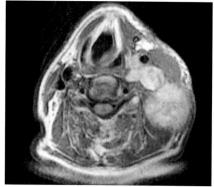

FIGURE 10.1A **FIGURE 10.1B**

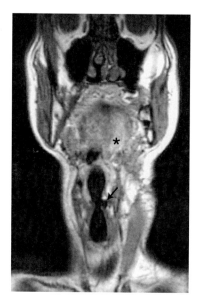

FIGURE 10.1C

CLINICAL HISTORY

An adult male with metastatic melanoma presents with persistent hoarseness.

FINDINGS

Axial T1-weighted image shows a left neck adenopathy. The left arytenoid cartilage is paramedian in position (Fig. 10.1A). The left true vocal cord is partially abducted and appears slightly inferior to that on the right. There is asymmetry on a higher section resulting from medial positioning of the left aryepiglottic fold and resultant widening of the left pyriform sinus (Fig. 10.1B). The coronal T1-weighted image confirms the inferior position of the sagging vocal cord and subsequent widening of the laryngeal ventricle (Fig. 10.1C). The tongue shows unilateral atrophy, suggesting a cranial nerve XII involvement.

DIAGNOSIS

Vocal cord paralysis.

DISCUSSION

Vocal cord paralysis may result from pathology in the brainstem, skull base, neck, or mediastinum. The recurrent laryngeal nerve innervates all the intrinsic muscles of the larynx. Paresis or palsy of this nerve usually results in a characteristic clinical and radiographic appearance of the larynx as well as hoarseness or weak voice. Because of the long course of the left recurrent laryngeal nerve, which loops around the ductus arteriosus before ascending up the tracheoesophageal groove to the vocal cord, it is particularly susceptible to injury.

The recurrent laryngeal nerve arises from the vagus nerve. The vagus nerve originates from the medulla and exits the skull base via the pars nervosa of the jugular foramen. It then travels inferiorly, just posterior to the carotid artery and jugular vein. Because of differences in vascular embryology between the two sides, the recurrent laryngeal nerve loops around the subclavian artery on the right and under the aortic arch (ductus arteriosus) on the left. Thus, imaging studies for right-sided disease only need to cover to the level of the subclavian artery, whereas evaluation of the left recurrent laryngeal nerve must cover sections down to the aortic arch. As with denervation elsewhere in the body, there is a subsequent laxity of the muscle groups following nerve injury. In the larynx, the most prominent muscle group is the thyroarytenoid muscle, which includes the vocalis muscle. Denervation results in medial rotation of the vocal process of the arytenoid cartilage and a paramedian position of the muscle, which may on radiographic studies simulate a small vocal cord mass. In addition, these structures also sag downward, causing ipsilateral widening of the laryngeal ventricle, which may be visible on coronal MRI. As the aryepiglottic fold is attached to the arytenoid cartilage, this downward displacement also results in ipsilateral widening of the pyriform sinus. These findings strongly suggest recurrent nerve paralysis and help distinguish this entity from other causes of vocal cord fullness.

With longstanding denervation, there may be atrophy as well as subtle fatty replacement visible as increased signal on MR T1-weighted images. There may also be increased signal on T2-weighted images unrelated to fatty replacement, which may be a change in water content related to loss of innervation.

Although recurrent laryngeal nerve dysfunction may be related to tumors or vascular conditions, or may be idiopathic, the vast majority of vocal cord paralysis is related to trauma during neck or thyroid surgery.

The superior laryngeal nerve exits the vagus nerve and innervates the cricothyroid muscle as well as providing sensory innervation of the larynx. It is usually not possible to diagnose this condition from the radiologic findings. However, because of subtle asymmetry of the larynx, the diagnosis may sometimes be made clinically with unilateral involvement. Imaging plays a role in this case in evaluating the course of the nerve from the larynx to the skull base to exclude pathology. With symmetric bilateral involvement, clinical or radiologic diagnosis is usually not possible. This usually causes adduction of the vocal cords and airway compromise, which helps to differentiate, vocal cord fullness due to paresis from other vocal cord masses.

The value of radiology in this condition is two-fold. First, the radiologist may suggest the diagnosis when the clinical picture is unclear and the imaging findings are characteristic. Second, once the diagnosis of laryngeal paralysis has been made, the entire course of the recurrent nerves from the brainstem to mediastinum must be evaluated for possible causes of dysfunction.

SUGGESTED READINGS

Decker GAG, du Plessis DJ. *Lee McGregor's synopsis of surgical anatomy,* 12th ed. Bristol: John Wright and Sons 1986;372.

Gacek M, Gacek RR. Cricoarytenoid joint mobility after chronic vocal cord paralysis. *Laryngoscope* 1996;106(12 Pt 1):1528–1530.

Jacobs CJ, Harnsberger HR, Lufkin RB, et al. Vagal neuropathy: evaluation with CT and MR imaging. *Radiology* 1987;164:97–102.

Tachimori Y, Kato H, Watanabe H, et al. Vocal cord paralysis in patients with thoracic esophageal carcinoma. *J Surg Oncol* 1995;59:230–232.

Tanaka S, Hirano M, Umeno H. Laryngeal behavior in unilateral superior laryngeal nerve paralysis. *Ann Otolrhinol-laryngol* 1994;103:93–97.

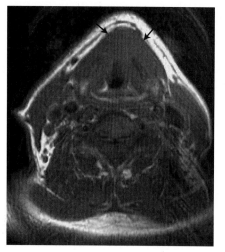

FIGURE 11.1A

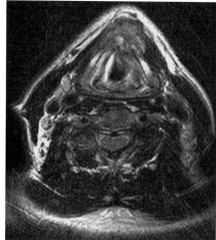

FIGURE 11.1B

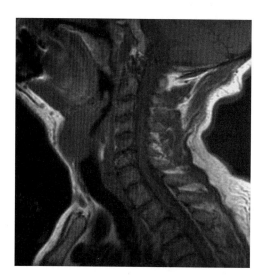

FIGURE 11.1C

CLINICAL HISTORY

A 47-year-old white male nonsmoker, social drinker, has a 2-year history of progressive hoarseness following an upper respiratory infection. Direct laryngoscopy revealed a necrotic-looking mass on the right vocal cord with extension across the anterior commissure to the left anterior cord. Subglottic extension was also noted.

FINDINGS

Axial T1-weighted images (Fig. 11.1A) through the larynx shows a large soft tissue mass with extension through the cartilage anteriorly into the soft tissues of the neck. The T2-weighted image better defines the tumor muscle contrast (Fig. 11.1B). The sagittal view shows that it extends from the supraglottis to the subglottis (Fig. 11.1C).

DIAGNOSIS

Transglottic squamous cell carcinoma of the larynx.

DISCUSSION

Most laryngeal malignancies are squamous cell carcinomas. The incidence is higher in men than in women and more common in middle-aged patients than in young patients. Smoking and/or alcohol are prominent risk factors in both sexes. Common presenting symptoms include hoarseness, cough, and dysphagia. Large tumors may cause airway compromise and lead to dyspnea.

Malignant laryngeal tumors are classified into three main subtypes by their anatomic location. Supraglottic tumors involve the laryngeal surface of the epiglottis, arytenoid cartilage, aryepiglottic folds, and false cords. Glottic tumors involve only the true cords. Subglottic tumors arise from structures below the inferior surface of the true cords. Transglottic tumors actually constitute a fourth subtype in which there is tumor extension across more than one anatomic subdivision. Midline ligaments tend to prevent tumor spread across the midline in all types of laryngeal cancer. Nodal involvement is usually unilateral.

By definition, transglottic carcinoma is a tumor that involves the true cord and false cord by crossing the laryngeal ventricle or the true cord and subglottic region. This crossing is frequently not seen by direct spread of the tumor from the true to false cord, or vice versa, but rather by invasion of the tumor deep to the mucosa in the paralaryngeal space, an area undetectable by direct visualization. Cord fixation usually means the cricoarytenoid joint is involved. Coronal or sagittal MR sections, being perpendicular to the vocal cords and laryngeal ventricles, can provide better delineation of tumor extension, sometimes underestimated on axial images.

Transglottic tumor, by crossing the laryngeal ventricle, as seen in this case, usually means that a total laryngectomy is to be performed, resulting in no natural speech conservation. Transglottic carcinoma of the larynx has a tendency to invade the thyroid cartilage, usually beneath the anterior commissure, and can extend beneath the cartilage to go through the cricothyroid membrane to involve the midline delphian nodes. Sagittal MR images of the midline would be best to detect involvement of this region.

SUGGESTED READINGS

Bailey BJ. Glottic carcinoma. In Bailey BJ, Biller HF, eds. *Surgery of the larynx.* Philadelphia: WB Saunders, 1985;257–278.

Batsakis JG. *Tumors of the head and neck: clinical and pathological considerations,* 2nd ed. Baltimore: Williams & Wilkins, 1979.

Castelijns JA, Geritsen GJ, Kaiser MC, et al. Invasion of laryngeal cartilage by cancer: comparison of CT and MR imaging. *Radiology* 1987;166:199–206.

Curtin HD. Imaging of the larynx: current concepts. *Radiology* 1989;173:1–11.

Lawson W, Biller HF. Glottic and subglottic tumors. In *Comprehensive management of the head and neck tumors.* Philadelphia: WB Saunders, 1987;991–1015.

Lufkin RB, Hanafee WN. Imaging of the laryngopharynx. *Semin US CT MR* 1986;7:166–180.

Lufkin RB, Hanafee WN, Wortham DG, et al. Larynx and hypopharynx: MR imaging with surface coils. *Radiology* 1986;158:747–754.

Mancuso AA, Hanafee WN. *Computer tomography and magnetic resonance imaging of the head and neck,* 2nd ed. Baltimore: Williams & Wilkins, 1985;241–357.

Teresi LM, Lufkin RB, Hanafee WN. Magnetic resonance imaging of the larynx. *Radiol Clin North Am* 1989;27:393–406.

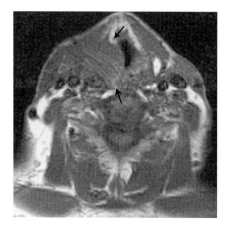

FIGURE 12.1A

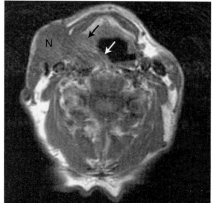

FIGURE 12.1B

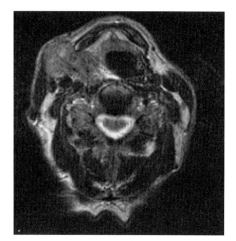

FIGURE 12.1C

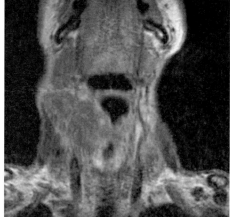

FIGURE 12.1D

CLINICAL HISTORY

A 62-year-old male complains of mild dysphagia of 6 weeks' duration.

FINDINGS

On axial T1-weighted images (Fig. 12.1A, B), a pyriform sinus mass is seen, well delineated from the surrounding fat. A large nodal metastasis is present. The tumor/muscle interface is indistinct. In contrast, on axial T2-weighted images (Fig. 12.1C), the high signal intensity of the tumor allows excellent differentiation from pharyngeal and prevertebral musculature but blends with fat. The coronal postcontrast image shows the craniocaudal extent of the mass (Fig. 1D).

DIAGNOSIS

Pyriform sinus carcinoma.

DISCUSSION

Pyriform sinus cancers behave more aggressively than endolaryngeal lesions and comprise 10% to 20% of "laryngeal" cancers. They are actually one of the most common cancers of the hypopharynx (posterior pharyngeal wall, pyriform sinuses, postcricoid region). They are usually advanced on presentation. Initial manifestations are often subtle and include pain in the throat or referred pain to the ear, with later dysphagia, otalgia, or an isolated lump in the neck. Unlike the hoarseness that occurs with vocal cord involvement, patients with pyriform sinus cancer often have a characteristic alteration in their vocalization described as a "potato voice." Early nodal disease occurs because of the rich lymphatics anterior to the pyriform sinuses.

Pathologically, the majority of these tumors are squamous cell carcinoma. They tend to spread submucosally, either (a) circumferentially with extension into the posterior pharyngeal wall or (b) posterolaterally with deep invasion and associated cartilage destruction. The size of the tumor does not necessarily relate to the degree of biologic aggressiveness or the tendency for cartilage destruction.

Pyriform sinus tumors grow in two major patterns:

1. Those of the lateral wall invade the thyroid cartilage and soft tissues of the neck, forming bulky masses about the pyriform sinus
2. Tumors of the medial wall extend into the paralaryngeal space and vocalis muscle, resembling marginal supraglottic lesions

Despite the similarities, pyriform sinus tumors have several characteristics that distinguish them from marginal supraglottic lesions. Pyriform sinus tumors frequently invade the thyroid cartilage, usually at its posterolateral margins. Also, pyriform sinus lesions tend to be unilateral and submucosal. If extensive, these tumors may widen the space between the thyroid and cricoid cartilages (cricothyroid notch). This is because the tough conus elasticus tends to direct the tumor posterolaterally and inferiorly.

Because clinical examination is often difficult and incomplete, cross-sectional imaging is necessary to evaluate the extent of submucosal spread. MR allows excellent soft tissue definition and is valuable in distinguishing tumor from surrounding structures. On T1-weighted images, the primary tumor signal intensity differs sufficiently from fat so that its margins are well seen. On T2-weighted images, the bright signal blends with fat but is clearly distinguished from surrounding musculature. Thus, T1-weighted sequences are better at determining tumor/fat contrast, whereas T2-weighted images are helpful in determining tumor/muscle contrast.

Surgical resection is the treatment of choice, often in conjunction with radiation therapy. Nodal dissection is performed as necessary.

SUGGESTED READINGS

Allal AS. Cancer of the pyriform sinus: trends towards conservative treatment. *Bull Cancer* 1997;84:757–762.
Elias MM, Hilgers FJ, Keus RB, et al. Carcinoma of the pyriform sinus: a retrospective analysis of treatment results over a 20-year period. *Clin Otolaryngol* 1995;20:249–253.
Larsson SV, Mancuso A, Hoover L, et al. Differentiation of pyriform sinus cancer from supraglottic laryngeal cancer by computed tomography. *Radiology* 1981;141:427–432.

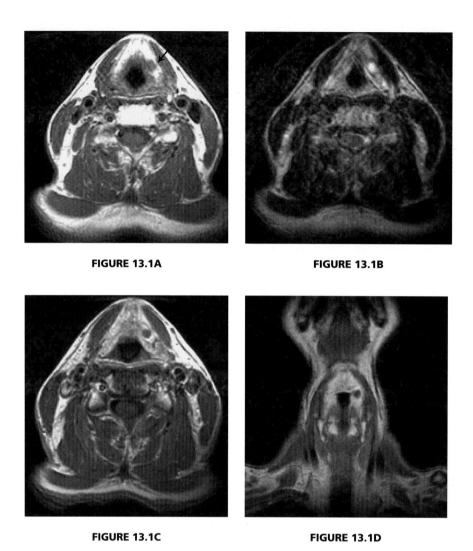

FIGURE 13.1A   FIGURE 13.1B

FIGURE 13.1C   FIGURE 13.1D

CLINICAL HISTORY

A 50-year-old male presents with hoarseness. On laryngoscopic examination there was a bulge in the false cord level.

FINDINGS

On the T1-weighted axial image, there is an oval, sharply marginated abnormality in the false cord obliterating the fat normally found there (Fig. 13.1A). The mucosa can be seen along the medial margin indicating that the lesion is in a submucosal position. The lesion is high signal intensity on T2-weighted images (Fig. 13.1B). On the postcontrast views, there is no evidence of enhancement (Figs. 13.1C, D).

DIAGNOSIS

Internal laryngocele.

DISCUSSION

Laryngoceles are formed by a dilation of the saccule (appendix) of the laryngeal ventricle. The laryngeal saccule is a small diverticulum that passes superiorly from the ventricle of the larynx. As such, it passes into the paraglottic space at the level of the false cord. Some authors use the term *saccular cyst* if it is fluid filled and *laryngocele* if it is air filled. More commonly, either form is referred to as a laryngocele.

When it expands superiorly in the paralaryngeal space, medial to the thyroid cartilage, it is known as an internal laryngocele and can present as a submucosal supraglottic space mass. Lateral displacement of the thyroid lamina can occur. Alternatively, if the dilated saccule extends through the thyrohyoid membrane out into the soft tissues of the neck, it is a mixed (external) laryngocele. This form may present as a soft tissue neck mass.

An unobstructed laryngocele is filled with air. With obstruction, high-protein fluid accumulates within the dilated appendix. If the obstructed fluid becomes infected, then it is referred to as a *pyolaryngocele.*

Laryngoceles are benign entities. Sometimes a small lesion (carcinoma) near the neck of the saccule causes the obstruction and subsequent formation of a laryngocele. The laryngeal saccule is normally collapsed, but if there is a tumor obstructing its outflow into the ventricle, it can dilate, forming a laryngocele or saccular cyst. Laryngoceles may also be associated with chronic granulomatous disease, such as tuberculosis.

The differential diagnosis of a submucosal mass in the larynx includes various benign and malignant lesions. Laryngoceles often have a unique imaging appearance that narrows the differential diagnosis. Laryngoceles are usually unilateral, although they may be bilateral in 25% of cases. Laryngoceles present commonly in adulthood; many are asymptomatic.

In imaging studies, a laryngocele is a rounded, well-circumscribed soft tissue mass or air collection that extends superiorly from the laryngeal ventricle and false cord into the paralaryngeal space (internal laryngocele) or lateral to the thyrohyoid membrane (mixed/external laryngocele). In mixed laryngoceles, both internal and external cystic features can be identified. The signal intensity of the fluid depends on the protein content.

A typical MR appearance depends on whether the laryngocele is filled with air or fluid. A signal void indicates that it is air filled, whereas the intermediate signal is consistent with a saccular cyst. The region of the ventricle should be carefully examined to exclude a tumor. Intravenous contrast may be helpful in defining the cystic nature of the lesion. Internal laryngoceles have been aspirated, incised, drained, and marsupialized. External/mixed laryngoceles are often treated via an external surgical approach following any internal components of the laryngocele for removal.

SUGGESTED READINGS

Curtin HD. Imaging of the larynx: current concepts. *Radiology* 1989;173:1–11.
Teresi LM, Lufkin RB, Hanafee WN. Magnetic resonance imaging of the larynx. *Radiol Clin North Am* 1989;27:393–406.

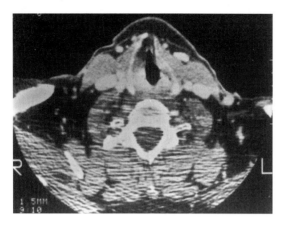

FIGURE 14.1A

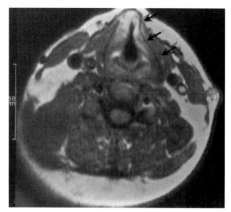

FIGURE 14.1B

CLINICAL HISTORY

A 61-year-old man complains of several weeks of weakness in his voice. He denies dysphagia and hoarseness but describes occasional pain in the laryngeal area on phonation. He does not drink alcohol or smoke and recalls no trauma to his neck.

Visualization of the larynx shows a submucosal mass in the region of the left false vocal cord.

FINDINGS

A CT scan at the level of the false vocal cords shows the laryngeal mass effect indenting the airway (Fig. 14.1A). No other soft tissue masses are noted.

Axial T1-weighted MRI at the same level also demonstrates the "mass" created by a low signal curvilinear structure (Fig. 14.1B).

DIAGNOSIS

Chronic posttraumatic deformity of the larynx.

DISCUSSION

Unlike acute laryngeal injury in which the history of trauma is usually the presenting finding, patients with chronic posttraumatic laryngeal deformities may present with a variety of vague symptoms and may deny any history of trauma.

Patients with chronic posttraumatic laryngeal deformities often present with asymptomatic, mucosal-covered laryngeal "masses" long after the initial (and often forgotten) trauma. Six factors are often found in the symptom complex of old laryngeal injury:

1. Voice fatigue
2. Sensation of food "sticking" in the throat

3. Soreness in the side of the neck
4. Submucosal mass in the supraglottic larynx
5. CT or MR evidence of trauma

Posttraumatic deformity of the laryngeal cartilages can be diagnosed by using CT and MRI. This is of particular aid to the clinician who is evaluating a laryngeal mass with no history of injury to the neck. CT and MRI are both effective in this situation, and, although MRI allows better soft tissue contrast resolution and can produce coronal and sagittal views, CT is probably superior for visualization of the ossified cartilage and associated changes.

The chronic findings of trauma of the larynx are soft tissue abnormalities caused by scarring and granulation, and posttraumatic deformity of the laryngeal skeleton. It is important to recognize the appearance of these chronic structural changes on the imaging studies because they may occur in individuals who do not recall the initial trauma.

Correct diagnosis may avoid an unnecessary biopsy or even more invasive procedures.

These patients usually need no specific management for the laryngeal deformity. If there is airway compromise or voice changes, specific therapy may be necessary.

SUGGESTED READINGS

Bent JP 3rd, Porubsky ES. The management of blunt fractures of the thyroid cartilage. *Otolaryngol Head Neck Surg* 1994;110:195–202.

Chui L, Lufkin R, Hanafee W. The use of MRI in the identification of post-traumatic laryngeal deformities. *Clin Imaging* 1990;14:127–130.

Hanson DG, Mancuso AA, Hanafee WN. Pseudomass lesions due to occult trauma of the larynx. *Laryngoscope* 1982;92:1249–1253.

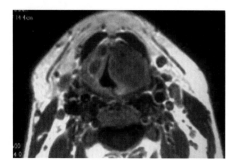

FIGURE 15.1A

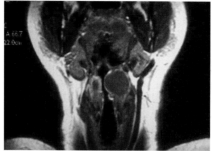

FIGURE 15.1B

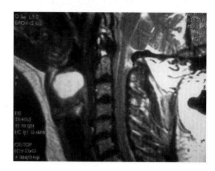

FIGURE 15.1C

CLINICAL HISTORY

A 49-year-old woman singer presents with progressive hoarseness and dyspnea.

FINDINGS

Axial T1-weighted images, coronal postcontrast T1-weighted images, and sagittal T2-weighted images (Figs. 15.1A–C) through the larynx show a large cystic, submucosal lesion in the supraglottic compartment extending superiorly along the left paraglottic space from the level of the laryngeal ventricle to the level of the petiole of the epiglottis. The lesion is pear-shaped, has well-defined linear enhancing borders, and causes stenosis of the laryngeal vestibule. On the contralateral side, a smaller similar lesion is seen in the same location with similar signal characteristics.

DIAGNOSIS

Bilateral fluid-filled laryngoceles.

DISCUSSION

Laryngoceles are benign acquired lesions resulting from an abnormal dilatation of the saccule or appendix, a small diverticulum of the laryngeal ventricle. Through a mechanism of increased glottic pressure or obstruction, this diverticulum may increase in size and extend superiorly along the paraglottic space, bulging the false vocal cords into the laryngeal vestibule. Laryngoceles have been associated with certain professions such as glass blowing, trumpet playing, and singing, which require repeated increases in endolaryngeal pressure, and with inflammatory or neoplastic conditions that may obstruct the saccule.

When confined to the endolaryngeal soft tissues, laryngoceles are classified as *internal*. However, continuing growth leads to a herniation of the laryngocele through the thyrohyoid membrane into the soft tissues of the lateral neck. These laryngoceles, with both internal and external components, are classified as *mixed type* and may present as a neck mass. Either type of laryngocele may be air or fluid filled. Air-filled laryngoceles have typical imaging findings and in most instances are not a diagnostic challenge. The only differential consideration is endolaryngeal emphysema resulting from mucosal disruption, usually in a posttraumatic or postintubation setting. Fluid-filled laryngoceles may mimic other cystic laryngeal or neck masses such as congenital laryngeal cysts, laryngeal mucoceles, vallecular cysts, and necrotic laryngeal neoplasms. Mixed laryngoceles may also mimic branchial cleft and thyroglossal duct cysts.

Congenital laryngeal cysts present in the pediatric age group with stridor and respiratory distress, and are epithelial-lined cysts with no connection to the laryngeal lumen. In the setting of hoarseness and a submucosal laryngeal mass seen endoscopically, imaging is helpful in establishing the diagnosis and in detecting any associated obstructive lesions of the laryngeal ventricle that may be responsible for the laryngocele formation.

On MR, fluid-filled laryngoceles are well-defined, pear-shaped lesions, usually following the signal intensity of cerebrospinal fluid (CSF) on all pulse sequences. When infected or inflamed, they may show linear marginal enhancement or T1-weighted hyperintensity as a result of high protein content or hemorrhage. Air-filled laryngoceles appear as flow voids.

Laryngoceles are managed surgically through incision, drainage, and marsupialization. Mixed laryngoceles with a large external component require an external surgical approach.

SUGGESTED READINGS

Carrat, X. Laryngomucocele as an unusual late complication of subtotal laryngectomy. Case report. *Ann Otol Rhinol Laryngol* 1998;107:703–707.

Castelijns JA. Imaging of the larynx. *Neuroimaging Clin N Am* 1996;6:401–415.

Chu L. Neonatal laryngoceles. A cause for airway obstruction. *Arch Otolaryngol Head Neck Surg* 1994;120:454–458.

Ingrams D. Laryngocele: an anatomical variant. *J Laryngol Otol* 1999;113:675–677.

Koeller KK. Congenital cystic masses of the neck: radiologic-pathologic correlation. *Radiographics* 1999;19:121–146; quiz 152–153.

Matino Soler E. Laryngocele: clinical and therapeutic study of 60 cases. *Acta Otorrinolaringol Esp* 1995;46:279–286.

Murray SP. Laryngocele associated with squamous carcinoma in a 20-year-old nonsmoker. *Ear Nose Throat J* 1994;73:258–261.

Sniezek JC. Laryngoceles and saccular cysts. *South Med J* 1996;89:427–430.

Thomas DM. Bilateral laryngoceles. *Ear Nose Throat J* 1993;72:819–21.

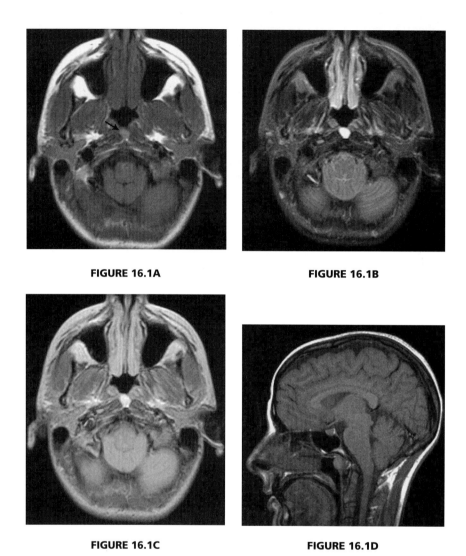

FIGURE 16.1A

FIGURE 16.1B

FIGURE 16.1C

FIGURE 16.1D

CLINICAL HISTORY

An adult man presents with headaches. A round, midline, mucosal-covered nasopharyngeal mass is noted. He denies foul breath, nasal discharge, or muscular spasm with head motion.

FINDINGS

A 5-mm homogeneously high signal intensity lesion on T1-weighted image (Fig. 16.1A), proton density image (Fig. 16.1B), and T2-weighted image (Fig. 16.1C) is present in the nasopharyngeal midline. The surrounding soft tissues are intact. The sagittal view reveals no intracranial communication (Fig. 16.1D).

DIAGNOSIS

Tornwaldt (or Thornwaldt) cyst.

DISCUSSION

Most Tornwaldt cysts are asymptomatic, with 4% being incidentally found at autopsies. When present, symptoms may include postnasal discharge, crusting, frequent colds, sneezing, hoarseness, bad taste or odor, coughing, or prevertebral neck pain with motion, nasal speech, cervical adenitis, or symptoms relating to the ear such as vertigo, tinnitus, earache, or deafness. With infection, prevertebral muscle spasm may occur.

The cyst develops in the region of the nasopharyngeal bursa, the site of the caudal-most end of the notocord, and results from an adhesion between the pharyngeal endoderm and the notocord. The bursa is more common in infants than in adults. The bursa may appear as a midline pit or may be closed over as a cyst.

The cyst, which may have a canal that extends to the pharyngeal mucosa, is situated beneath the adenoid, or its remnants, and extends backward and upward to the periosteum of the occipital bone. This canal may become obstructed, resulting in infection and abscess formation.

Tornwaldt cysts vary from 1 to 5 mm in diameter and are generally rounded. They may, on rare occasions, extend off the midline. They usually are fluid filled but occasionally they contain air. MRI demonstrates high signal intensity both on T1-weighted and T2-weighted images, likely related to either proteinaceous or hemorrhagic cyst contents. The integrity of the overlying bone should always be confirmed with sagittal, coronal, or more cephalad axial views in order to rule out the rare meningocele or encephalocele.

Treatment for symptomatic lesions includes surgical drainage and excision.

SUGGESTED READINGS

Ikushima I, Korogi Y, Makita O, et al. MR imaging of Tornwaldt's cysts. *AJR Am J Roentgenol* 1999;172:1663–1665.
Miyahara H, Matsunaga T. Tornwaldt's disease. *Acta Otolaryngol Suppl* 1994;517:36–39.

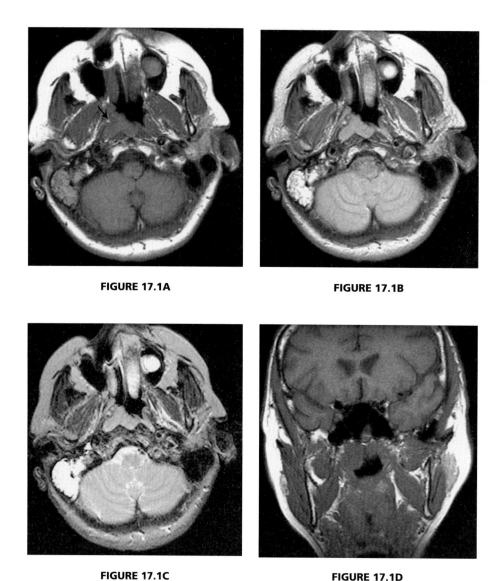

FIGURE 17.1A

FIGURE 17.1B

FIGURE 17.1C

FIGURE 17.1D

CLINICAL HISTORY

A 50-year-old woman presents with a history of progressive hearing loss on the right side.

FINDINGS

A T1-weighted axial sequence of the nasopharynx shows diffuse soft tissue infiltration of the vault of the right nasopharynx with low to intermediate signal on T1-weighted images. There is obliteration of the fossae of Rosenmüller as well as ipsilateral opacification of the mastoid air cells (Fig. 17.1A). Extension of this lesion beyond the pharyngobasilar fascia is present, indicating an aggressive lesion. The proton density–weighted image improves the tumor muscle contrast (Fig. 17.1B). The T2-weighted image shows similar findings (Fig. 17.1C). The mass in the left maxillary sinus is a retention cyst. The coronal T1-weighted image shows no evidence of skull base invasion (Fig. 17.1D).

DIAGNOSIS

Non-Hodgkin's lymphoma of the nasopharynx.

DISCUSSION

Non-Hodgkin's lymphoma is the second most common histologic diagnosis (after squamous carcinoma) made in nasopharyngeal malignancies. The lesion usually appears smooth, exophytic, submucosal, and nonulcerative. Extranodal lymphoma in the head and neck region increases the probability of systemic disease below the clavicle or diaphragm, and the majority of patients have involvement of cervical lymph nodes. The tonsils are most often involved, followed by the nasopharynx and the lymphoid tissue of the base of the tongue.

In the nasopharynx, symptoms related to the ear usually lead to early detection of the tumor when it is fairly small because of the proximity of the lesion to the orifice of the eustachian tube.

The majority of cases of extranodal lymphomas of the head and neck are histiocytic lymphomas and lymphocytic lymphomas of the diffuse type. Involvement of extranodal sites of the head and neck by Hodgkin's disease is rare. Most of the patients with lymphoma limited to the head and neck are in the fourth to eighth decades of life.

The pharyngobasilar fascia is the superior fascial continuation of the constrictor muscles of the pharynx. It separates the pharyngeal mucosa from the deeper musculature and holds the airway open as it attaches to the skull base. It is composed of the deep layer of the deep cervical fascia.

On MR or contrast-enhanced CT scanning, it can often be identified by its "whale tail" configuration, which provides an important imaging landmark to help differentiate benign from more aggressive nasopharyngeal masses. Normal adenoidal lymphoid tissue does not cross this boundary, whereas malignancies such as carcinoma and lymphoma and aggressive infections do. Lymphoma of the nasopharynx may be indistinguishable on imaging studies from nasopharyngeal carcinoma. A bulky and diffuse nasopharyngeal mass with extensive adenopathy should suggest the diagnosis. Similar findings (nasopharynx mass and adenopathy) may be seen with human immunodeficiency virus–positive patients and in younger patients with infectious mononucleosis.

Radiation therapy and chemotherapy are the primary modes of treatment for lymphoma.

SUGGESTED READINGS

Braun IF. MRI of the nasopharynx. *Radiol Clin North Am* 1989;27:327.

Kieserman SP, Stern J. Malignant transformation of nasopharyngeal lymphoid hyperplasia. *Otolaryngol Head Neck Surg* 1995;113:474–476.

Yanagisawa E, Citardi MJ. Endoscopic view of malignant lymphoma of the nasopharynx. *Ear Nose Throat J* 1994;73:514–516.

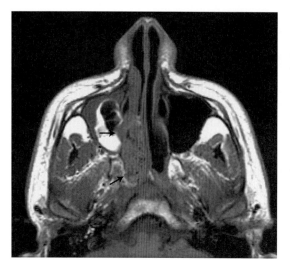

FIGURE 18.1A

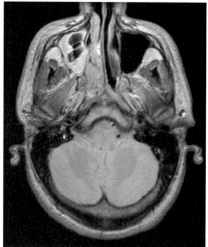

FIGURE 18.1B

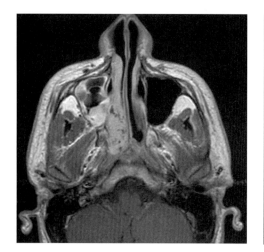

FIGURE 18.1C

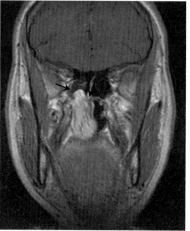

FIGURE 18.1D

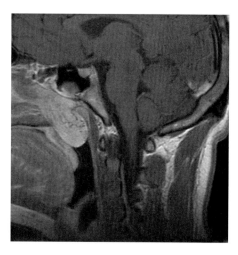

FIGURE 18.1E

CLINICAL HISTORY

A teenaged male complains of nasal stuffiness for 1 year and several episodes of spontaneous nose bleeds for 6 months.

FINDINGS

The axial T1-weighted image shows a mass in the right posterior nasal cavity and nasopharynx (Fig. 18.1A). The T2-weighted image shows areas of flow void within the mass. The adjacent maxillary sinus shows inflammatory change (Fig. 18.1B). The postcontrast image shows uniform enhancement of the mass (Fig. 18.1C). The coronal postcontrast image shows invasion of the floor of the sphenoid sinus (Fig. 18.1D). The sagittal image confirms these findings (Fig. 18.1E).

DIAGNOSIS

Juvenile nasopharyngeal angiofibroma (JNA).

DISCUSSION

Juvenile nasopharyngeal angiofibroma is a benign tumor of the nasopharynx composed of fibrous connective tissue and an abundance of endothelium-lined vascular spaces. The name of the disease is derived from the fact that it occurs during adolescence, almost exclusively in boys. The most common presenting complaint is nasal obstruction and epistaxis.

Although the pathogenesis is not fully understood, the tumor is thought to be a malformation of vascular tissue. These tumors are believed to originate in the posterolateral wall of the nasal cavity near or within the sphenopalatine foramen. JNAs tend to follow vessels as they grow through natural foramina and fissures, expanding as they grow. The vascular supply is primarily via branches of the external carotid artery. The angiographic appearance is characteristic. With intracranial extension, the internal carotid artery may also supply portions of the mass. Extension may commonly be found in the infratemporal fossa (via the pterygomaxillary fissure), orbital apex (via the inferior orbital fissure), sphenoid sinus, and, less often, into the middle cranial fossa via foramen rotundum.

The punctate and serpentine areas of signal void seen on MR suggest a highly vascular lesion. Widening of the pterygopalatine fossa is perhaps the most helpful distinguishing feature of JNAs (occurring in more than three fourths of patients in one study). CT optimally demonstrates the bony changes, usually with remodeling and thinning of bone without frank destruction. Diagnostic angiograms are no longer routinely done. Preoperative embolization is performed on almost all lesions. Accurate radiologic diagnosis is important because biopsy of a JNA can lead to severe hemorrhage.

Surgery is the treatment of choice for these lesions with preoperative embolization in nearly all cases. Radiation therapy is used in selected cases that are not amenable to surgical resection.

SUGGESTED READINGS

Antonelli AR, Cappiello J, Di Lorenzo D, et al. Diagnosis, staging, and treatment of juvenile nasopharyngeal angiofibroma. *Laryngoscope* 1987;97:1319–1325.

Brooker DS, Kenny B, Gibson RG, et al. Juvenile nasopharyngeal angiofibroma in a static population: the implications of misdiagnosis. *Clin Otolaryngol* 1989;14:497–502.

Economou TS, Abemayor E, Ward PH. Juvenile nasopharyngeal angiofibroma: an update of the UCLA experience, 1960–1985. *Laryngoscope* 1988;98:170–175.

Jamal MN. Imaging and management of angiofibroma. *Eur Arch Otorhinolaryngol* 1994;251:241–245.

Lloyd GA, Phelps PD. Juvenile angiofibroma: imaging by magnetic resonance, CT and conventional techniques. *Clin Otolaryngol* 1986;11:247–259.

Ungkanont K, Byers RM, Weber RS, et al. Juvenile nasopharyngeal angiofibroma: an update of therapeutic management. *Head Neck* 1996;18:60–66.

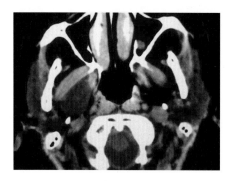

FIGURE 19.1A   **FIGURE 19.1B**

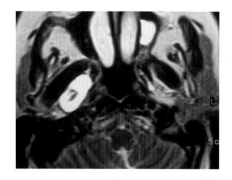

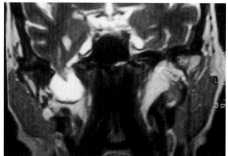

FIGURE 19.2A   **FIGURE 19.2B**

CLINICAL HISTORY

A 67-year-old woman undergoes a brain CT for headaches and dizziness.

FINDINGS

Axial postcontrast CT section through the maxillary antra (Fig. 19.1A) shows a well-defined cystic mass in the right infratemporal fossa (masticator space) between the external and internal pterygoid muscles.

Another section (Fig. 19.1B) at the level of the skull base shows that the mass communicates with the intracranial compartment through a defect in the greater wing of the sphenoid bone at the level of the foramen ovale.

Axial T2-weighted MR sections (Fig. 19.2A) show that the lesion is not purely cystic, having a solid component at the level of the sphenoidal bony defect. Coronal T2-weighted image (Fig. 19.2B) shows that the solid component of the lesion is a portion of the left anterior temporal lobe herniating through the bony defect covered by meninges with an associated meningocele filled with cerebrospinal fluid (CSF).

DIAGNOSIS

Trans-sphenoidal cephalocele.

DISCUSSION

Cephaloceles belong to a spectrum of congenital anomalies related to closure of the anterior neuropore during embryologic development. Bony defects of the skull base or skull vault occur when rests of ectoderm become entrapped, leading to failure of mesodermal ingrowth. Subsequently, a variety of embryologic defects ranging from herniation of intracranial contents to nasal gliomas, dermoids and epidermoid cysts, and sinus tracts may occur.

Cephaloceles are classified according to their contents and location. *Meningocele* is the term used when there is only herniation of the meninges, and *cephalomeningoceles* is the term used when, in addition, they contain brain tissue. Depending on their location, cephaloceles are classically subdivided into *occipital,* the most common, *sincipital,* located in the anterior skull and presenting with an external mass, and *basal* cephaloceles, located at the skull base and not visible externally unless large enough to protrude into a natural orifice (usually the nasal or oral cavities). Basal cephaloceles may occur trough transethmoidal, trans-sphenoidal, sphenoethmoidal, and frontosphenoidal defects and most often they are clinically occult and remain unrecognized until adulthood.

Although most cephaloceles are diagnosed immediately after birth or in the pediatric age group (85%), some come to clinical attention or are incidental imaging findings during adulthood. These may be a diagnostic challenge and have disastrous outcomes when misdiagnosed. Patients with idiopathic CSF fistulas or repeated bouts of meningitis should undergo a workup for congenital or acquired skull defects.

MR is the modality of choice because it clearly demonstrates the contents of the herniated tissue (meninges, CSF, and brain parenchyma) and, because of its multiplanar capability, localizes the bony defect. Although invasive, high-resolution CT with thin sections and bone algorithm after intrathecal injection of myelographic contrast can also be used. Imaging may detect associated bony anomalies of the skull or facial bones. Surgical correction is advised to prevent complications.

SUGGESTED READINGS

Ayadi K, Trans-ethmoid encephaloceles. *J Radiol* 1999;80:558–590.

Fitzpatrick E, Miller RH. Congenital midline masses: dermoids, gliomas and encephaloceles. *J Louisiana State Med Soc* 1996;148:93–96.

Kanonier GJ. Congenital intranasal cephalocele: diagnosis and treatment. *Acta Otorhinolaryngol Ital* 1996;16:441–446.

Martinez-Lage JF. The child with a cephalocele: etiology, neuroimaging and outcome. *Childs Nerv Syst* 1996;12:540–550.

Martinez-Lage JF. Craniosynostosis in neural tube defects: a theory on its pathogenesis. *Surg Neurol* 1996;46:465:9; discussion 469–470.

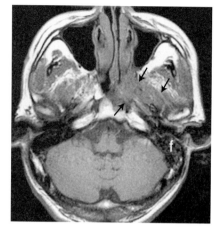

FIGURE 20.1A

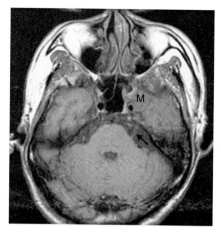

FIGURE 20.1B

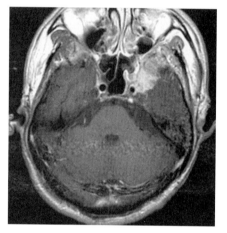

FIGURE 20.1C

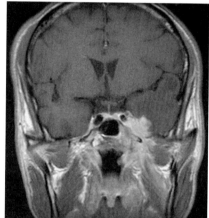

FIGURE 20.1D

CLINICAL HISTORY

A 42-year-old man has unilateral serous otitis media.

FINDINGS

Axial T1-weighted images show fluid in the left mastoid. There is also a mass in the left nasopharynx extending laterally (Fig. 20.1A). The next higher section shows a mass in Meckel's cave and lateral displacement of the cisternal portion of the left trigeminal nerve (Fig. 20.1B). The postcontrast T1-weighted view at the same level shows uniform enhancement of the mass (Fig. 20.1C). The coronal enhanced T1-weighted image shows the nasopharyngeal mass extending upward through foramen ovale toward Meckel's cave (Fig. 20.1D).

DIAGNOSIS

Squamous cell carcinoma of the nasopharynx.

DISCUSSION

The nasopharynx remains an area that is occult to casual clinical examination. Its proximity to the skull base makes cancers in this region particularly devastating. Malignancies of the nasopharynx can be divided into three groups: (a) 70% are carcinomas, (b) 20% are lymphomas, and (c) the remaining 10% are made up of a variety of lesions including adenocarcinoma, rhabdomyosarcoma, melanoma, adenoid cystic carcinoma, and others.

Carcinoma of the nasopharynx is classified according to the World Health Organization based on histopathology into three types. Type I (20%) is *keratinizing squamous cell carcinoma*, which is similar to other lesions found in the upper aerodigestive system. Type II lesions (30%) have little or no keratin production and are referred to as *nonkeratinizing carcinoma*. Because of their similarity to urinary tract tumors, they are sometimes referred to as transitional cell carcinomas. Type III carcinomas are *undifferentiated* (50%). The 5 year survival rate for types I, II, and III is typically around 20%, 40%, and 60%, respectively. Whereas type I and II lesions are usually found in adults, type III lesions have a bimodal age distribution.

Whereas carcinoma of the nasopharynx is an uncommon tumor in the United States, in certain portions of the world (e.g., Canton, China) it is one of the most common cancers. Human leukocyte antigen A2 and B-sin histocompatibility loci have been identified as possible markers in the Chinese population for susceptibility to this disease. Even though the incidence of the disease in American born Chinese decreases, it is still seven times higher than for other Americans.

Antibodies against Epstein-Barr virus have been associated with the undifferentiated form of nasopharyngeal carcinoma. Other risk factors for nasopharyngeal carcinoma include exposure to nitrosamines (found in dry, salted fish), aromated hydrocarbons (found in burned foods), and nickel.

Nasopharyngeal carcinoma may present as a change in voice quality, impaired hearing, or a mass in the nasopharynx. Often the first sign of abnormality is the accumulation of fluid in the middle ear or mastoid caused by obstruction of the eustachian tube.

Lymphadenopathy is also very common in nasopharyngeal carcinoma and is seen in approximately 70% of patients at presentation. Nodal extension to the nodes of Rouviere (lateral retropharyngeal nodes) is frequent. A common presentation of nasopharyngeal carcinoma is a mass in the nasopharynx and cervical lymphadenopathy.

MR examination of the nasopharynx is indicated to:

1. Delineate the extent of a known malignancy.
2. Search for the presence of the tumor in a patient with symptoms or clinical findings.
3. Follow up patients who have undergone treatment for nasopharyngeal cancer to rule out recurrence.

Anatomic routes by which tumors extend from the nasopharynx to the middle cranial fossa may be shown by imaging studies. By following the eustachian tube, nasopharyngeal carcinoma can pass through the tough pharyngobasilar fascia at its only natural defect, the sinus of Morgagni. From this point, a tumor may enter the parapharyngeal space and extend to the floor of the middle cranial fossa by extending along the course of the eustachian tube in the sphenoidal sulcus, following it to the region of the foramen lacerum and ovale, and then extending into the cavernous sinus. Tumors high in the nasopharynx may also gain access to the middle cranial fossa via either the pterygoid canal or sphenopalatine foramen. Through the pterygoid canal, tumors may extend directly to the foramen lacerum or erode through the thin lateral wall of sphenoid sinus, entering the cavernous sinus. Through the sphenopalatine foramen, tumors may extend directly to the pterygopalatine fossa, inferior and superior orbital fissures, and into the cavernous sinus. In cases of nasopharyngeal carcinoma with neck metastases, MR images may show extranodal tumor abutting and surrounding the carotid artery and jugular vein.

The role of surgery in this disease is limited to biopsy and staging. Radiation therapy is the standard treatment for nasopharyngeal carcinoma. The addition of chemotherapy is becoming the standard of care for this disease.

SUGGESTED READINGS

Teresi LM, Lufkin RB, et al. MR imaging of the nasopharynx and floor of the middle cranial fossa. Part I. Normal anatomy. *Radiology* 1987;164:811.

Teresi LM, Lufkin RB, et al. MR imaging of the nasopharynx and floor of the middle cranial fossa. Part II. Malignant tumors, etc. *Radiology* 1987;164:817.

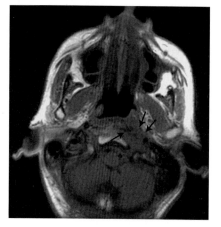

FIGURE 21.1A

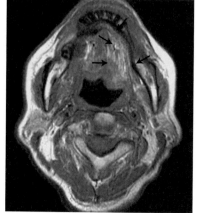

FIGURE 21.1B

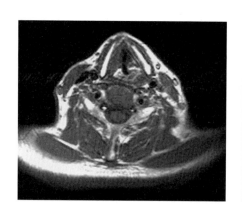

FIGURE 21.1C

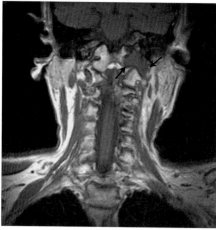

FIGURE 21.1D

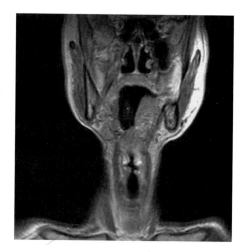

FIGURE 21.1E

CLINICAL HISTORY

A 40-year-old man with a history of nasopharyngeal carcinoma presents with new hoarseness and tongue fullness.

FINDINGS

The axial T1-weighted MR image (Fig. 21.1A) shows fullness in the right nasopharynx with a mass that extends to the ipsilateral hypoglossal canal. The lower axial T1-weighted image through the tongue shows increased bulk on the right with higher signal intensity and atrophy of the tongue musculature (Fig. 21.1B). The axial T1-weighted image through the true vocal cords shows a paramedian position of the cord on the right (Fig. 21.1C). The postcontrast coronal T1-weighted image again shows the skull base mass (Fig. 21.1D). The more anterior coronal image shows the right tongue fullness and the inferior position of the right true vocal cord (Fig. 21.1E).

DIAGNOSIS

Squamous cell carcinoma of the nasopharynx with extension to the skull base resulting in hypoglossal and recurrent laryngeal nerve palsies.

DISCUSSION

See related discussions of nasopharyngeal carcinoma, hypoglossal palsy, and recurrent nerve (vocal cord) palsy.

SUGGESTED READINGS

Batchelor TT, Krol GS, DeAngelis LM. Neuroimaging abnormalities with hypoglossal nerve palsies. *J Neuroimaging* 1996;6:240–242.

Jacobs CJ, Harnsberger HR, Lufkin RB, et al. Vagal neuropathy: evaluation with CT and MR imaging. *Radiology* 1987;164:97–102.

King AD, AhuJa A, Leung SF, et al. MR features of the denervated tongue in radiation induced neuropathy. *Br J Radiol* 1999;72:349–353.

Russo CP, Smoker WR, Weissman JL. MR appearance of the trigeminal and hypoglossal motor denervation. *AJNR Am J Neuroradiol* 1997;18:1375–1383.

Tanaka S, Hirano M, Umeno H. Laryngeal behavior in unilateral superior laryngeal nerve paralysis. *Ann Otol Rhinol Laryngol* 1994;103:93–97.

Teresi LM, Lufkin RB, et al. MR imaging of the nasopharynx and floor of the middle cranial fossa. Part II. Malignant tumors, etc. *Radiology* 1987;164:817.

Teresi LM, Lufkin RB, et al. MR imaging of the nasopharynx and floor of the middle cranial fossa. Part I. Normal anatomy. *Radiology* 1987;164:811.

Thompson EO, Smoker WR. Hypoglossal nerve palsy: a segmental approach. *Radiographics* 1994;14:939–958.

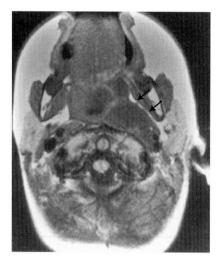

FIGURE 22.1A

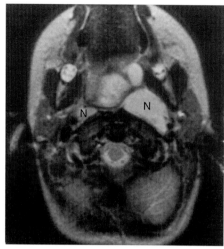

FIGURE 22.1B

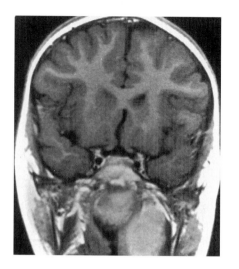

FIGURE 22.1C

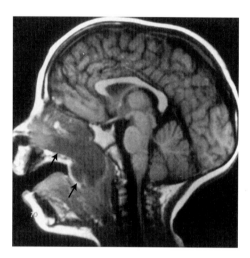

FIGURE 22.1D

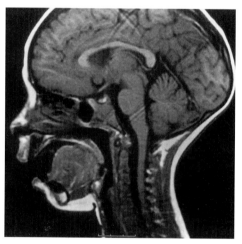

FIGURE 22.1E

CLINICAL HISTORY

A 3-year-old girl presents with history of chronic nasal obstruction.

FINDINGS

Axial T1-weighted MR images show an enhancing lobulated soft tissue mass occupying most of the posterior and left lateral aspect of the oropharynx and nasopharynx, extending anteriorly into the nasal cavity and inferiorly to the oropharynx (Fig. 22.1A). Axial T2-weighted images show a clear separation between the primary mass and bilateral retropharyngeal nodal conglomerates, most prominent on the left side (Fig. 22.1B). Coronal enhanced T1-weighted MR image shows the craniocaudal extent of the mass and homogeneous contrast enhancement (Fig. 22.1C). There is no evidence of meningeal spread or intracranial invasion through the cranial nerves foramina (Fig. 22.1C). Sagittal T1-weighted MR image shows a bulky soft tissue mass occupying the nasopharynx, nasal cavity, nasal vault, and oropharynx, obstructing the choana and oropharyngeal airway (Fig. 22.1D). Sagittal T1-weighted MR image (same patient after radiotherapy and chemotherapy) shows complete resolution of the soft tissue mass (Fig. 22.1E).

DIAGNOSIS

Nasopharyngeal rhabdomyosarcoma (embryonal type).

DISCUSSION

Rhabdomyosarcoma is the most common malignant soft tissue tumor in children younger than 15 years of age. In the head and neck, it is the most common sarcoma and the third most common malignancy following lymphoma and retinoblastoma. Two peaks of prevalence are noted, one between 2 and 5 years of age and the other between 15 and 20 years. Seventy percent of tumors present before age 10. In the head and neck, the most common location is the orbit, followed in decreasing order of frequency by the nasopharynx, paranasal sinuses, and middle ear cavity.

Rhabdomyosarcoma is a malignant mesenchymal tumor that originates from undifferentiated mesenchymal cells, precursors of skeletal muscle. No predisposing factors are recognized, but a chromosomal translocation is noted in almost half of the children with rhabdomyosarcoma. Pathologically, three main types of spindle cell tumor are recognized. The most common is the embryonal type, which comprises 75% of all cases and is the form most commonly encountered in the head and neck. This cell type is seen in younger children and carries a better prognosis, with a 5-year survival rate of 65% after combined treatment with radiotherapy and chemotherapy. Histologically, the embryonal cell type may be confused with anaplastic carcinoma, large cell lymphoma, esthesioneuroblastoma, and melanoma. Botryoid rhabdomyosarcoma is not histologically different from the embryonal type, and its name is derived from its macroscopic grapelike appearance. The second most common, the alveolar type (15%), tends to occur in older patients (second decade), spreads to lymph nodes, and carries a worse prognosis, with only a 2% 5-year survival rate. Finally, the least common form is pleomorphic rhabdomyosarcoma, which is considered to be an adult form because only 6% of cases occur before age 6 years.

Clinical presentation depends on the location of the tumor. Nasopharyngeal rhabdomyosarcomas tend to grow silently and present as large destructive masses at a late stage. Very young children may have difficulty breathing and eating, and failure to thrive. Older children present with sinonasal symptoms similar to those of sinus infection, which further delays the diagnosis. Nasal obstruction, rhinorrhea, and epistaxis are the most common presenting symptoms. Hearing impairment as a result of obstructive serous otitis is also common. Local pain appears late in the course of the disease and usually indicates bony destruction. Cranial nerve and other neurologic signs and symptoms imply skull base invasion with intracranial extension.

Overall, lymph node metastasis is seen in 50% of cases at presentation and distant metastasis in 58%. The most common metastatic sites include the lungs, bone marrow, and brain.

Imaging is crucial for the diagnosis, determination of local and distant tumor extent, treatment planning, and detection of local recurrence.

Cross-sectional imaging may disclose the aggressive nature of a nasopharyngeal mass by showing deep invasion and bone destruction, which cannot be assessed on clinical examination, differentiating adenoidal hypertrophy from more aggressive lesions. However, lack of specificity in tissue characterization necessitates biopsy to confirm the diagnosis.

MRI is the modality of choice in evaluation of soft tissue

tumors of the head and neck. It allows multiplanar delineation of tumor, differentiation between tumor and postobstructive inflammatory changes, and detection of meningeal and cranial nerve spread in postcontrast images.

Rhabdomyosarcoma tends to be of intermediate signal intensity on T1-weighted images and hyperintense on T2-weighted images, and it enhances homogeneously. Cervical and retropharyngeal lymphadenopathy should be surveyed. It has been demonstrated that the presence of a post-therapeutic residual mass, defined as a region of soft tissue thickening at the original tumor site with enhancement and absence of mass effect, is a poor prognostic sign, heralding an increased probability of tumor recurrence.

The overall prognosis of rhabdomyosarcoma markedly improved with the advent of multidrug chemotherapeutic regimens and external beam radiotherapy, from a 55% to an 80% 5-year survival rate in patients with nonmetastatic disease. These regimens had their major impact in the treatment of parameningeal tumors not amenable to curative surgery or requiring major craniofacial resections with inadequate surgical margins. Surgery plays an important role in many patients.

SUGGESTED READINGS

Gilles R, Couanet D, Sigal R, et al. Head and neck rhabdomyosarcomas in children: value of clinical and CT findings in the detection of loco-regional relapses. *Clin Radiol* 1994;49:412–415.

Kowalski LP, San CI. Prognostic factors in head and neck soft tissue sarcomas: analysis of 128 cases. *J Surg Oncol* 1994;56:83–88.

Kraus DH, Saenz NC, Gollamudi S, et al. Pediatric rhabdomyosarcoma of the head and neck. *Am J Surg* 1997;174:556–560.

Lee JH, Lee MS, Lee BH, et al. Rhabdomyosarcoma of the head and neck in adults: MR and CT findings. *AJNR Am J Neuroradiol* 1996;17:1923–1928.

Lyos AT, Goepfert H, Luna MA, et al. Soft tissue sarcoma of the head and neck in children and adolescents. *Cancer* 1996;77:193–200.

Odell PF. Head and neck sarcomas: a review. *J Otolaryngol* 1996;25:7–13.

Park YW. Evaluation of neck masses in children. *Am Fam Phys* 1995;51:1904–1912.

Yang WT, Kwan WH, Li CK, et al. Imaging of pediatric head and neck rhabdomyosarcomas with emphasis on magnetic resonance imaging and a review of the literature. *Pediatr Hematol Oncol* 1997;14:243–257.

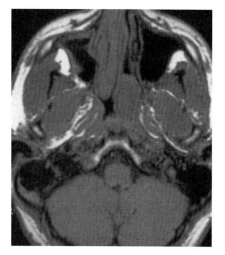

FIGURE 23.1

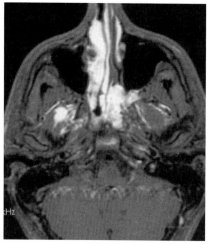

FIGURE 23.2

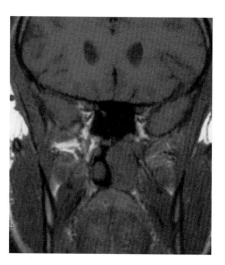

FIGURE 23.3

CLINICAL HISTORY

A 19-year-old male has a 1-year history of recurrent epistaxis and nasal obstruction. He was found to have a nasopharyngeal mass. He denied visual changes, facial numbness or pain, and dysphasia.

FINDINGS

A well-defined soft tissue mass is seen in the left nasopharynx extending to the posterior left nasal cavity (Fig. 23.1). The lesion is markedly enhanced following contrast administration (Fig. 23.2) with suggestion of several foci of flow void. The lesion clearly extends to the left pterygopalatine fossa (Fig. 23.3). Preoperative angiogram shows numerous feeding vessels to the nasopharyngeal mass from the sphenopalatine artery, accessory meningeal artery, and ascending palatal artery (not shown). No feeding vessels are seen from the internal carotid artery in this case.

DIAGNOSIS

Juvenile nasopharyngeal angiofibroma (JNA).

DISCUSSION

JNA is a benign hypervascular tumor that occurs almost exclusively in teenaged males. The most common presenting complaints are nasal obstruction and recurrent epistaxis. These tumors are believed to originate from the sphenopalatine foramen, which is the medial exit of the pterygopalatine fissure. From there, it usually spreads to the nasopharynx, posterior nasal cavity, infratemporal fossa via the pterygomaxillary fissure, and intracranial compartment via the foramen rotundum or inferior orbital fissure. The posterior wall of the maxillary sinus is usually bowed forward. JNAs are a benign but locally aggressive tumor, and they tend to follow vessels as they grow through natural foramina and fissures. The staging system developed by Chandler et al. is as follows:

Stage I: Tumor limited to the nasopharynx
Stage II: Extension into the nasal cavity and/or sphenoid sinus

Stage III: Extension into the maxillary or ethmoid sinuses, pterygomaxillary or infratemporal fossa, orbit, or cheek

Stage IV: Intracranial extension

The vascular supply is primarily supplied by branches of the internal maxillary artery (sphenopalatine and descending palatine branches) and ascending pharyngeal artery. Once the lesion grows, the blood supply from branches of the facial or ophthalmic artery (ethmoid branches) or internal carotid artery (vidian artery, meningo-hypophyseal artery, or inferolateral trunk) can be seen. Preoperative embolization of the feeding vessels is help-ful to reduce amount of hemorrhage associated with surgery.

Classic MR appearance of JNA is abundance of flow voids from its high vascularity. A soft tissue mass in the nasopharynx or posterior nasal cavity with involvement of pterygopalatine fissure and sphenopalatine foramen in a teenaged male with epistaxis is fairly diagnostic. The angiomatous polyp in the nasal cavity may have a similar radiographic and clinical presentation and should be considered if the patient is female or an older male. The other potential differential diagnosis should include rhabdomyosarcoma, schwannoma of the trigeminal nerve, and nasopharyngeal carcinoma.

SUGGESTED READINGS

Antonelli AR, Cappiello J, Di Lorenzo D, et al. Diagnosis, staging, and treatment of juvenile nasopharyngeal angiofibroma. *Laryngoscope* 1987;97:1319–1325.

Chandler JR, Goulding R, Moskowitz L, et al. Nasopharyngeal angiofibroma: staging and management. *Ann Otol Rhinol Laryngol* 1984;93:322–329.

Economou TS, Abemayor E, Ward PH. Juvenile nasopharyngeal angiofibroma: an update of the UCLA experience, 1960–1985. *Laryngoscope* 1988;98:170–175.

Gullane PJ, Davidson J, O'Dwyer T, et al. Juvenile angiofibroma: a review of the literature and case series report. *Laryngoscope* 1992;102:928–933.

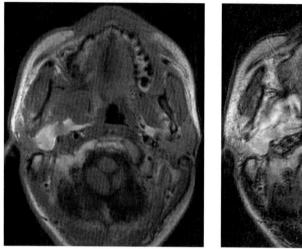

FIGURE 24.1A

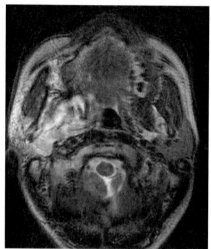

FIGURE 24.1B

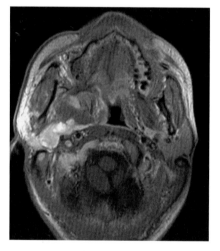

FIGURE 24.1C

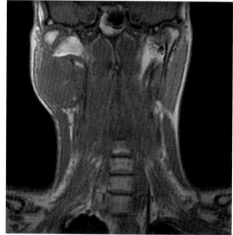

FIGURE 24.1D

CLINICAL HISTORY

A 64-year-old woman presents with a mass in the right lateral neck. On physical examination, a soft, nontender, mobile mass was palpated underneath the right mandibular angle and in the right submandibular region.

FINDINGS

Axial T1-weighted MR image of the neck shows a high signal mass centered in the right prestyloid parapharyngeal space (PPS) contiguous with the deep lobe of the parotid (Fig. 24.1A). Medially, it slightly bulges the right lateral wall of the oropharynx. This well-defined lesion causes mass effect but does not appear to infiltrate the adjacent structures. The signal follows that of the subcutaneous fat on the remainder of the images (Fig. 24.1B–D).

DIAGNOSIS

PPS liposarcoma.

DISCUSSION

Lipomatous lesions in the PPS present as any other mass in the same location. They cause few, if any, symptoms until they become large and compress adjacent neurovascular structures or compromise the airway.

Earaches, tubal dysfunction, and fullness or foreign body sensation in the oropharynx may be the presenting symptoms and are nonspecific. When large enough, these lesions may cause airway obstruction. When palpable, they manifest as soft, lobulated masses that may or may not be mobile. Differential diagnosis of a PPS mass includes abscess, atypical branchial cleft cyst, benign and malignant salivary gland rest tumors, mesenchymal tumors, such as lipoma and hemangioma, and, less commonly, neural sheath tumors.

Fatty tumors are common in the body, but only 13% occur in the head and neck region. In the head and neck, they can be subcutaneous or submucosal, and the most common location is in the subcutaneous soft tissues of the posterior neck. They tend to grow with age and are more common in obese people. Although they enlarge with increasing body weight, they do not decrease in size with weight loss.

Liposarcomas are much less common than lipomas and are exceedingly rare in the head and neck. The ratio of liposarcoma-to-lipoma has been estimated as 1:20. The incidence of liposarcomas above the clavicles is low, approximately 5%, and there are only 80 cases described in the literature. There is a slight male predominance with a male-to-female ratio of 3:2. The age range is broad, with a peak incidence in the sixth decade.

Liposarcomas are malignant tumors that arise from lipoblasts or totipotential mesenchymal cells, usually adjacent to muscle or fascia. They are much more common in the deep-seated fat, rarely arising in the subcutaneous soft tissues. They do not originate from preexisting lipomas.

The histologic classification of these tumors is controversial in that the biologic behavior of adipose tissue neoplasms depends not only on morphology but also on location. According to some authors, fatty neoplasms arising in deep fatty spaces tend to behave in a more aggressive fashion than their histologic counterparts in subcutaneous fat. Therefore, deep adipose tissue neoplasms should be considered malignant even in the absence of cytologic features of malignancy.

Depending on their histologic features, liposarcomas are usually classified into four categories: well-differentiated, myxoid, round cell, and pleomorphic. Whereas the former two categories rarely metastasize and have a high 5-year survival rate, the latter show a high recurrence rate and a high rate of distant metastasis.

Imaging is crucial in the diagnosis of lesions seated in the deep spaces of the neck, which are not accessible to clinical examination. It is not uncommon for a PPS mass to be detected as an incidental finding in a study performed for unrelated reasons.

Both CT and MRI are well suited to detect masses in the PPS and may be diagnostic when a lipomatous lesion is seen. Although the imaging appearance of lipomatous tumors is characteristic on CT scans, liposarcomas may be difficult or impossible to diagnose based on imaging because they may mimic any other soft tissue tumor (malignant fibrous histiocytoma, lymphoma, plasmocytoma, rhabdomyosarcoma). Depending on their histologic subtype, they may contain varying amounts of fat intermingled with other soft tissue components. Therefore, the density of the lesion depends on its composition and vascularity, and may be similar to that of muscle.

The MRI appearance of liposarcomas in the head and neck is not well documented because of the rarity of this entity. However, it has been reported that the appearance of liposarcomas differs from subcutaneous fat in that the signal characteristics of fat within a liposarcoma tends to be of lower signal intensity on T1-weighted sequences and of higher signal intensity on T2-weighted sequences.

MRI is less specific than CT in diagnosing fatty tumors because the signal characteristics may overlap with those of mature hematomas. Several techniques have been used to separate these entities, including calculation of T1-weighted and T2-weighted relaxation times, gradient echo imaging, and several techniques of fat suppression. However, even using these techniques, a definite diagnosis is not always possible because hemorrhage within a fatty lesion is not infrequent. The most reliable technique to detect fat on MRI is frequency selective fat suppression imaging (FATSAT) in which a specific saturation pulse in the resonant frequency of fat is given.

Advantages of MRI in the evaluation of liposarcomas include a better delineation of the neoplasm and demonstration of the presence or absence of cleavage planes between the tumor and adjacent structures, as a result of its multiplanar capability.

Metastatic lymphadenopathy is infrequently seen.

Liposarcomas of the head and neck should be managed surgically by wide local excision. In the PPS, several approaches can be used depending on the size of the lesion and the surgeon's preference. These include transcervical, submandibular, transparotid, transoral, and infratemporal approaches. In selected cases, adjuvant radiotherapy may be of benefit. Palliative radiation therapy may prolong survival in inoperable cases. Neck dissections are not performed routinely because cervical metastasis is rare.

SUGGESTED READINGS

Abdullah BJ, Liam CK, Kaur H, et al. Parapharyngeal space lipoma causing sleep apnoea. *Br J Radiol* 1997;70:1063–1065.

Collins MH, Chatten J. Lipoblastoma/lipoblastomatosis: a clinicopathologic study of 25 tumors. *Am J Surg Pathol* 1997;21:1131–1137.

Elango S. Parapharyngeal space lipoma. *Ear Nose Throat J* 1995;74:52–53.

Kraus MD, Guillou L, Fletcher CD. Well-differentiated inflammatory liposarcoma: an uncommon and easily overlooked variant of a common sarcoma. *Am J Surg Pathol* 1997;21:518–527.

Saddik M, Oldring DJ, Mourad WA. Liposarcoma of the base of tongue and tonsillar fossa: a possibly underdiagnosed neoplasm. *Arch Pathol Lab Med* 1996;120:292–295.

Stewart MG, Schwartz MR, Alford BR. Atypical and malignant lipomatous lesions of the head and neck. *Arch Otolaryngol Head Neck Surg* 1994;120:1151–1155.

CASE 25

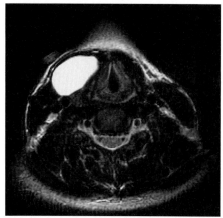

FIGURE 25.1A

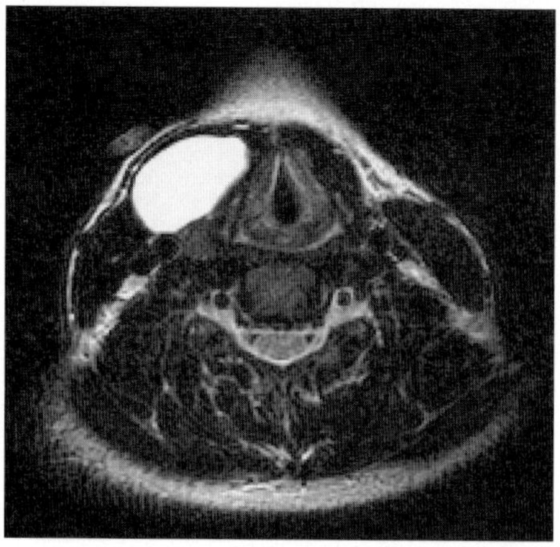

FIGURE 25.1B

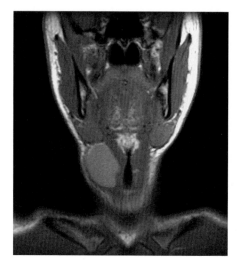

FIGURE 25.1C

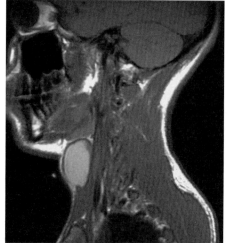

FIGURE 25.1D

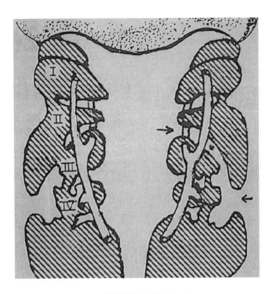

FIGURE 25.2

CLINICAL HISTORY

An adult male presents with a history of progressive swelling in his neck. Physical examination reveals a round, painless mass just inferior to the right submandibular gland.

FINDINGS

Axial MR shows there is a well-circumscribed thin-walled cystic mass in the right lateral neck (Fig. 25.1A). It is bright on T2-weighted image (Fig. 25.1B). The submandibular gland and larynx are normal. The mass is anterior to the sternocleidomastoid muscle and carotid artery and jugular vein. The coronal and sagittal images show similar findings (Fig. 25.1C, D).

DIAGNOSIS

Second branchial cleft cyst.

DISCUSSION

The second branchial cleft cyst most often presents as a smooth, nontender, fluctuant mass located along the upper third of the sternocleidomastoid muscle. When not in communication with an external fistula, the cyst may go unnoticed until the second to fourth decades. The discovery of the cyst is often related to an upper respiratory infection, which causes transient enlargement of the cyst. The cyst may become infected and progress to abscess formation, with the possibility that spontaneous rupture or incision and drainage will lead to a permanent fistula. Patients with a branchial fistula may present with persistent mucus discharge from a skin opening in the neck.

Second branchial cleft cysts are the most common con-genital cystic neck masses. Second branchial cleft anomalies comprise a spectrum of cysts, sinus tracts, and fistulas that are caused by incomplete obliteration of the branchial apparatus. The branchial apparatus begins to develop in the third week of gestation, surrounding the primitive pharynx and consisting of five transverse mesodermal ridges, separated by clefts. Each cleft is met by an outpouching of the pharynx, the pharyngeal pouch, with a thin membrane separating the structures at their interface. The branchial apparatus develops into the main structures of the face, nasopharynx, oropharynx, and neck.

The second branchial arch forms, among other structures, the styloid process, anterior base of the tongue, and posterior belly of the digastric muscle. The fate of the second branchial cleft is controversial, but in conjunction with remnants of the second pharyngeal pouch, it is believed to be responsible for 95% of branchial cleft cysts.

Second branchial cleft cysts occur via the persistence of the cleft as an epithelium-lined tract that courses between the second and third branchial arch (Fig. 25.2). If the tract exists in its entirety, that is, if there is a complete fistula, its internal opening usually lies in the tonsillar fossa. From there, the tract runs beneath the stylohyoid muscle and posterior belly of the digastric muscle and above the glossopharyngeal and hypoglossal nerves. Further on, it crosses between the internal and external carotid arteries. Below the carotid bifurcation, it courses along the carotid sheath anteromedial to the sternocleidomastoid muscle. The external opening appears along the anterior edge of the sternocleidomastoid, usually in its middle third. If the tract is incomplete, it may present as an isolated cyst anywhere along the course of the tract or as a cyst in communication with an internal or external fistula.

On CT and MR, a branchial cleft cyst often presents as an oval, well-defined, cystic mass near the mandibular angle with displacement of the sternocleidomastoid posteriorly and the carotid and jugular vein posteromedially. The cyst may insinuate between the internal and external carotid arteries. This appearance is pathognomonic.

On MRI, a noninfected second branchial cleft cyst presents as a well-circumscribed, thin-walled, homogeneously low to intermediate signal intensity cystic mass on T1-weighted images, and is usually high signal intensity on T2-weighted images. Varying degrees of wall thickening and increased T2-weighted signal intensity and obliteration of the surrounding fat planes may be seen if there has been previous infection.

Differential diagnosis may include neck abscess, infective or inflammatory lymphadenopathy (especially tuberculous adenitis), cystic hygroma, thyroglossal duct cyst, thymic cyst, laryngocele, paraganglioma, branchiogenic carcinoma, lipoma, and metastatic neoplasm. The benign, thin-walled, cystic appearance, the classic location, and the T1 and T2 parameters usually allow the correct imaging diagnosis.

Complete excision is the treatment of choice with low overall recurrence rate.

SUGGESTED READINGS

Agaton-Bonilla FC, Gay-Escoda C. Diagnosis and treatment of branchial cleft cysts and fistulae. A retrospective study of 183 patients. *Int J Oral Maxillofac Surg* 1996;25:449–452.

Androulakis M, Johnson JT, Wagner RL. Thyroglossal duct and second branchial cleft anomalies in adults. *Ear Nose Throat J* 1990;69:318–322.

Ford GR, Balakrishnan A, Evans JN, et al. Branchial cleft and pouch anomalies. *J Laryngol Otol* 1992;106:137–143.

Kenealy JF, Torsiglieri AJ Jr, Tom LW. Branchial cleft anomalies: a five-year retrospective review. *Trans Pennsylvania Acad Ophthalmol Otolaryngol* 1990;42:1022–1025.

Koeller KK, Alamo L, Adair CF, et al. Congenital cystic masses of the neck: radiologic-pathologic correlation. *Radiographics* 1999;19:121–146; quiz 152–153.

Reynolds JH, Wolinski AP. Sonographic appearance of branchial cysts. *Clin Radiol* 1993;48:109–110.

Roback SA, Telander RL. Thyroglossal duct cysts and branchial cleft anomalies. *Semin Pediatr Surg* 1994;3:142–146.

Todd NW. Common congenital anomalies of the neck. Embryology and surgical anatomy. *Surg Clin North Am* 1993;73:599–610.

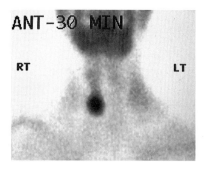

FIGURE 26.1A

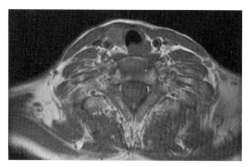

FIGURE 26.1B

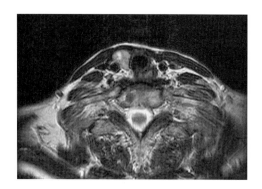

FIGURE 26.1C

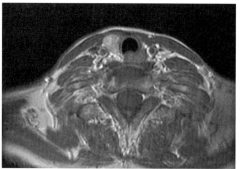

FIGURE 26.1D

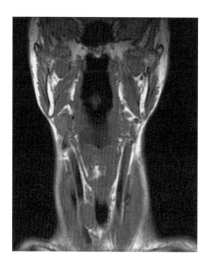

FIGURE 26.1E

CLINICAL HISTORY

A 50-year-old woman post-thyroidectomy presents with fatigue, weakness, and diffuse bone pain. Biochemical analysis showed hypercalcemia.

FINDINGS

Tc-Sestamibi scan shows increased uptake in the right thyroid bed on the right (Fig. 26.1A). Axial T1-weighted MRI shows a well-circumscribed rounded mass along the right aspect of the trachea (Fig. 26.1B). The normal thyroid gland is not visible on these images. The T2-weighted image shows increased signal in the mass (Fig. 26.1C). On postcontrast images, there is uniform enhancement (Fig. 26.1D). Coronal views confirm these findings (Fig. 26.1E). No lymphadenopathy is seen.

DIAGNOSIS

Parathyroid adenoma.

DISCUSSION

Primary hyperparathyroidism has a prevalence of 0.037%, with 100,000 new cases diagnosed annually in the United States. The disease is more prevalent in postmenopausal women with a peak incidence between the fifth and sixth decades. It results from increased secretion of parathyroid hormone (PTH) and subsequent hypercalcemia. Parathyroid adenoma accounts for most of the cases of primary hyperparathyroidism (80% to 85%), followed by parathyroid hyperplasia (15%), parathyroid cysts (<5%), and parathyroid carcinoma (<1%). Multiple adenomas are present in less than 5% of cases. Ectopic adenomas are not uncommon, representing 10% of all cases.

To localize the lesion, it is important to know the anatomy and embryology of the parathyroid glands. Normally, four parathyroid glands are present in each individual (two superior and two inferior), but supernumerary glands, up to six in number, are seen in 13% of people. The superior parathyroids originate from the endoderm of the fourth pharyngeal pouch along with the thyroid gland. Because their descent to normal position is minimal and intimately related to the thyroid gland, their position behind the upper lower third of the thyroid is relatively constant. Ectopic locations include (a) at or above the superior thyroid pole, (b) posterior and medially in the retropharyngeal region, and (c) below the inferior thyroid artery. Mediastinal locations are rare and are usually in the posterior mediastinum.

The inferior parathyroid glands originate from the third pharyngeal pouch in close relation to the thymic anlage. Because the glands migrate a long distance along with the thymus, ectopic locations are more frequent (50%). The most common anatomic location for the inferior parathyroid glands is lateral to the lower pole of the thyroid. Ectopic locations may be anywhere from the angle of the mandible to the low anterior mediastinum. Intrathyroid and intrathymic locations are seen in 2% of cases.

The optimal imaging modality for assessment of primary hyperparathyroidism and whether imaging is necessary in all patients are topics of debate. Because the diagnosis is usually made on the basis of clinical and biochemical data, the primary role of imaging is to localize the disease preoperatively and to detect any other head and neck pathology that may be treated simultaneously. However, because most parathyroid adenomas are perithyroidal in location, surgical treatment alone without preoperative localization is successful in 70% to 90%, depending on the series and experience of the surgical team. Although preoperative imaging improves this success rate to 97%, opponents of this approach argue that it does not significantly change surgical morbidity or operative time. Also, some studies suggest that the cost of preoperative imaging outweighs its benefits. Arguments to support preoperative imaging include the need for only unilateral cervicotomy when a single adenoma is detected, identification of ectopic adenomas, and reduction in operating room time. Therefore, the approach should be tailored to each particular institution depending on the experience of both the head and neck surgeon and radiologist and the availability of imaging modalities.

The options for imaging the parathyroid glands are multiple and include ultrasound, CT, MRI, and nuclear medicine studies. Studies comparing the accuracy of these imaging modalities alone and in several different combinations show conflicting results in different series. Far from being consensual, general guidelines suggest the use of a functional study (parathyroid scintigraphy) in association with an anatomic study (cross-sectional imaging). In the newly diagnosed patient, ultrasound should be used as the screening modality because it is the least expensive and most widely available of all modalities, followed by MRI when the results are negative or doubtful. The approach for residual and recurrent hyperparathyroidism includes MRI and parathyroid scintigraphy. For difficult, conflicting cases, intraoperative ultrasound and invasive studies, such as angiography and venous sampling for PTH levels, are recommended.

MRI is the most accurate of the cross-sectional modalities in detecting eutopic or ectopic parathyroid adenomas. These lesions are of intermediate signal intensity on T1-weighted image and hyperintense on T2-weighted image, and they show intense, homogeneous enhancement in most cases. However, highly cellular lesions may be of higher signal intensity on T1-weighted image and show intermediate signal intensity on T2-weighted image as a result of low water content. The most common MRI pitfall is confusion with an enlarged lymph node.

Parathyroid adenomas can be heterogeneous with areas of cystic degeneration and hemorrhage, causing further con-fusion with exophytic thyroid lesions. Calcification of a parathyroid adenoma is, however, uncommon. Concomitant thyroid lesions are seen in 41% of patients with primary hyperparathyroidism. Ill-defined margins, invasion of adjacent structures, and the presence of cervical lymphadenopathy are all suggestive of malignancy.

The gold standard for treatment of parathyroid adenoma is surgical resection. When a single lesion is successfully localized preoperatively, a unilateral cervicotomy is performed. However, some authors recommend intraoperative determination of PTH levels to exclude the possibility of a second missed lesion. When no presurgical imaging is performed, bilateral cervicotomies are routinely performed, and, if no lesions are found, an anterior cervicotomy or mediatinostomy may be required. For high surgical risk patients or patients who refuse surgery, parathyroid adenomas may be managed by image-guided therapies such as ethanol ablation, laser ablation, or electrocautery.

SUGGESTED READINGS

Hodin RA, Silen WW. Detection and management of parathyroid tumors. *Curr Opin Oncol* 1997;9:75–78.
Hopkins CR, Reading CC. Thyroid and parathyroid imaging. *Semin Ultrasound CT MR* 1995;16:279–295.
Loevner LA. Imaging of the parathyroid glands. *Semin Ultrasound CT MR* 1996;17:563–575.
Norton JA. Reoperation for missed parathyroid adenoma. *Adv Surg* 1997;31:273–297.
Santos E, Higgins CB, Clark O. Clinical image. Recurrent hyperparathyroidism caused by a parathyroid cystic adenoma: localization by MRI. *J Comput Assist Tomogr* 1996;20:996–998.
Yousem DM, Scheff AM. Thyroid and parathyroid gland pathology. Role of imaging. *Otolaryngol Clin North Am* 1995;28:621–649.

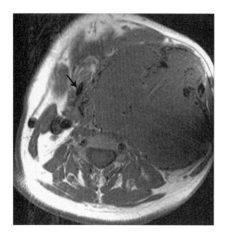

FIGURE 27.1A

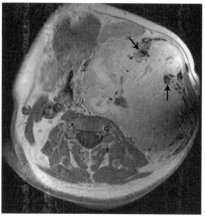

FIGURE 27.1B

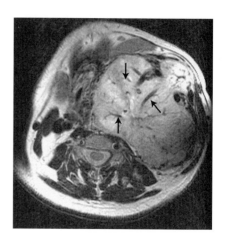

FIGURE 27.1C

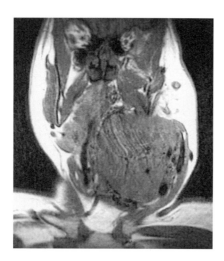

FIGURE 27.1D

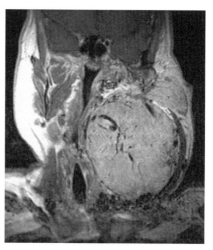

FIGURE 27.1E

CLINICAL HISTORY

A 56-year-old man presents with a left neck mass.

FINDINGS

The axial T1-weighted image shows a left-sided mass centered in the bifurcation of the carotid arteries (Fig. 27.1A) displacing the airway. The postcontrast T1-weighted image shows that the carotid arteries are splayed by the mass (Fig. 27.1B). The T2-weighted shows multiple serpentine flow voids within the mass (Fig. 27.1C). The coronal views precontrast and postcontrast show similar findings (Fig. 27.1D, E).

DIAGNOSIS

Massive left carotid body tumor.

DISCUSSION

A paraganglioma is a slowly growing neuroendocrine endoplasm that arises from neural crest derivatives. Chemodectoma, glomus tumor, nonchromaffin paraganglioma, and neurocristopathic tumor are the most common names given to this lesion. The precapillary arteriovenous shunts and nonchromaffin cells are characteristic of the histologic appearance of these tumors.

Paragangliomas can be classified by their locations, which can be tympanic and jugular. These tumors are less frequent and their clinical manifestations are similar, so they are usually classified as a single entity: temporal or jugulotympanic paragangliomas. Tumors of carotid and vagal locations are more frequent, with almost one half arising in the temporal bone. Paragangliomas are the most common neoplasms in the middle ear and are second in frequency to neurogenic tumors in the temporal bone.

There is a tendency of multicentricity of tumors (10%), especially in a patient with a carotid body tumor showing familial tendency (26%). The incidence of true malignancy showing metastasis is higher in a carotid body tumor (10%) than the overall incidence, varying from 2% to 6%. The biologic behavior or natural course of the tumors is not clearly correlated with histologic appearances.

The clinical findings of paragangliomas are slowly growing and compressible masses or cranial nerve paralysis, according to the location. In a temporal lesion, conductive or sensorineural hearing loss or pulsatile tinnitus may be the initial symptom, and a vertically fixed and laterally movable mass is a characteristic finding in a carotid body tumor.

Radiologic diagnosis of this tumor is based on the location of tumor and characteristic hypervascularity. For evaluation of the temporal bone, thin-slice, high-resolution CT is the imaging modality of choice; however, in other locations, MRI has some advantages in delineating and characterizing the lesion with its superb soft tissue contrast. The hypervascular nature of the tumor can be demonstrated by MR with signal void of flowing vessel.

Surgery is the therapy of choice for most patients with single lesions. Although conventional angiography is generally no longer used for diagnosis, preoperative embolization is used in most cases to limit bleeding at surgery. Radiation therapy is used in some patients who are not surgical candidates.

SUGGESTED READINGS

Bastounis E, Maltezos C, Pikoulis E, et al. Surgical treatment of carotid body tumours. *Eur J Surg* 1999;165:198–202.

Larson TC II, Reese DF, Baker HL Jr, et al. Glomus tympanicum chemodectomas: radiographic and clinical characteristics. *Radiology* 1987;163:801–806.

Netterville JL, Reilly KM, Robertson D, et al. Carotid body tumors: a review of 30 patients with 46 tumors. *Laryngoscope* 1995;105:115–126.

Olsen WL, Dillon WP, Kelly WM, et al. MR imaging of paragangliomas. *AJNR Am J Neuroradiol* 1986;7:1039–1042.

Rodraiguez-Cuevas S, Laopez-Garza J, Labastida-Almendaro S. Carotid body tumors in inhabitants of altitudes higher than 2000 meters above sea level. *Head Neck* 1998;20:374–378.

Shugar MA, Mafee MF. Diagnosis of carotid body tumors in dynamic computerized tomography. *Head Neck Surg* 1982;4:518–521.

Som PM, Sacher M, Stollman AL, et al. Common tumor of the parapharyngeal space: refined imaging diagnosis. *Radiology* 1988;169:81–85.

Vogl T, Bruning R, Schedel H, et al. Paragangliomas of the jugular bulb and carotid body: MR imaging with short sequences and GD-DTPA enhancement. *AJNR Am J Neuroradiol* 1989;10:823–827.

Win T, Lewin JS. Imaging characteristics of carotid body tumors. *Am J Otolaryngol* 1995;16:325–328.

Zak FG, Lawson W. *The paraganglionic chemoreceptor system. Physiology, pathology, and clinical medicine.* New York: Springer-Verlag, 1982:267–285.

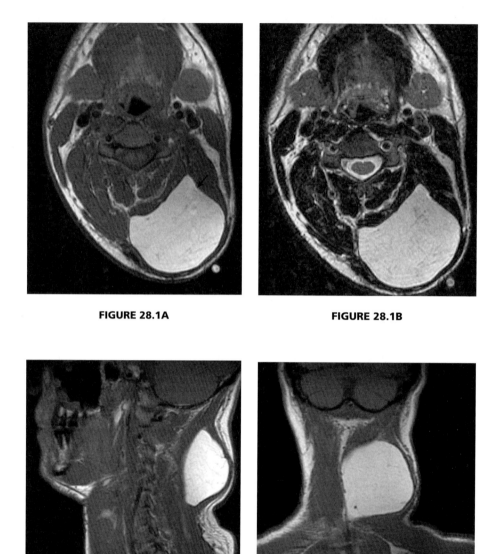

FIGURE 28.1A   **FIGURE 28.1B**

FIGURE 28.1C   **FIGURE 28.1D**

CLINICAL HISTORY

An adult male presents with a painless mass in the left posterior neck. On examination, a soft, mobile mass is palpated.

FINDINGS

Axial MRI of the neck shows a large, well-circumscribed mass in the subcutaneous tissues of the left posterior neck (Fig. 28.1A). The signal intensity of the mass follows fat on all pulse sequences (Fig. 28.1B–D).

DIAGNOSIS

Posterior neck lipoma.

DISCUSSION

Thirteen percent of lipomas occur in the head and neck, most commonly in the posterior neck subcutaneous tissues. Lipomas in the submucosa of the pharynx and larynx have been reported but are rare. Patients usually present for cosmetic reasons and rarely with compressive symptoms.

Lipomas are delicately encapsulated benign mesenchymal tumors of mature adipose tissues. Numerous microscopic subtypes have been described. Fibrolipomas have fat cells separated into lobules by septa of connective tissues. Angiolipomas, rare in the head and neck, are highly vascularized and may infiltrate adjacent muscles and neuromuscular bundles. Spindle cell lipomas are characterized by a mixture of fat cells and spindle-shaped fibroblasts in a collagenous matrix. These tumors appear more aggressive and may be confused with well-differentiated liposarcomas. Submucosal lipomas may arise within a muscle or from intermuscular fascial septa. These deeply seated lipomas may be sessile or pedunculated.

The unique characteristics of fat on both CT and MRI allow for the imaging diagnosis of most lipomas. On CT, lipomas are well-defined, noncontrast enhancing, with fat attenuation of -65 to -130 HU. A thin, smooth capsule and internal septations may be seen. On MRI, lipomas follow the signal characteristics of fat, which is hyperintense on T1-weighted image and intermediate on T2-weighted image. When the diagnosis is in doubt, additional fat suppression sequence may be performed.

Treatment is by surgical excision when warranted. There appears to be a high rate of recurrence, up to 62%, believed to be secondary to microscopic foci of lipomatous infiltration of adjacent soft tissues. Liposuction-assisted excision of lipomas may be used in cervicofacial lesions to improve the cosmetic result. The technique can be reperformed as needed in case of recurrence, with no significant increase in surgical risks. Submucosal lesions, depending on their size and location, may be removed endoscopically or via an external approach.

SUGGESTED READINGS

Calhoun KH, Bradfield JJ, Thompson C. Liposuction-assisted excision of cervicofacial lipomas. *Otolaryngol Head Neck Surg* 1995;113:401–403.

Eckel HE, Jungehülsing M. Lipoma of the hypopharynx: preoperative diagnosis and transoral resection. *J Laryngol Otol* 1994;108:174–177.

Kransdorf MJ. Benign soft-tissue tumors in a large referral population: distribution of specific diagnoses by age, sex, and location. *AJR Am J Roentgenol* 1995;164:395–402.

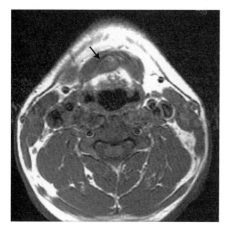

FIGURE 29.1A

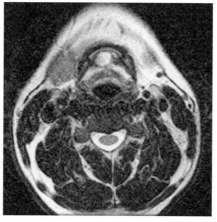

FIGURE 29.1B

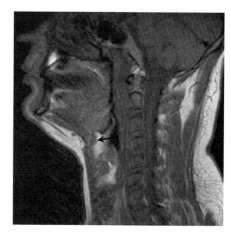

FIGURE 29.1C

CLINICAL HISTORY

The patient has painless midline swelling adjacent to the hyoid bone.

FINDINGS

Axial MR scans show a small rounded mass adjacent to the hyoid bone (Fig. 29.1A). On T2-weighted images, it appears to be cystic and have thin walls (Fig. 29.1B). The sagittal view shows that there is no significant craniocaudal extension (Fig. 29.1C).

DIAGNOSIS

Thyroglossal duct cyst.

DISCUSSION

The thyroglossal duct is an epithelial lined tubular structure extending from the foramen cecum, around the inferior border of the hyoid bone to the pyramidal lobe of the thyroid bed. It is formed by the third week of gestation and normally involutes by the tenth week. If any portion fails to involute, the secretory epithelial lining may cause a cyst to be formed. Although these are congenital lesions, they often do not present until there is inflammation or blockage of drainage.

Most patients have painless neck masses within the anterior triangle. Fistulas are uncommon but can occur related to surgery or complicated infection. Most cysts (>75%) are midline and are most common at or near the level of the hyoid bone.

Thyroglossal duct cysts are frequently found in children but they may also present in adulthood. They can be found anywhere along the thyroglossal tract, extending from the foramen cecum to the thyroid gland, and most frequently present as anterior, midline, or paramedian neck masses. They may be seen as a mass of the root of the tongue. The cyst is often associated with the body of the hyoid bone, and in order to avoid a surgical recurrence, it should be removed along with the body of the hyoid bone.

Thyroglossal duct cysts typically appear as a cystic, thin-walled midline mass on CT or MR scanning. They may be intimately associated with the hyoid bone. Thyroglossal duct cysts appear on CT as well-circumscribed fluid-density structures in the midline.

On MRI, the fluid contents demonstrate the same anatomic and gross morphologic features. Cyst fluid shows both long T1 and T2 in appropriately weighted spin echo images. The signal of the fluid depends on its contents (e.g., protein, hemorrhagic fluid). The cyst rim is nonenhancing on CT or MRI unless inflammation is present, which is often the case on symptomatic lesions. Perhaps the most significant morphologic feature to be determined by CT or MRI is whether there is evidence of internal or external fistulas, adherence to underlying structures, or lobulations, because these seem to be the most important causes of surgical recurrences.

Surgery is the treatment of choice. The goal is to remove all the epithelial lining. Because of their extent, complete removal may be difficult and recurrences may occur. Extensive resection (Sistrunk procedure), which removes the entire duct, midportion of the hyoid bone, and a portion of the tongue base, has decreased the recurrence rate significantly.

SUGGESTED READINGS

Kawanaka M, Sugimoto Y, Suehiro M, et al. Thyroid imaging in a typical case of acute suppurative thyroiditis with abscess formation due to infection from a persistent thyroglossal duct. *Ann Nucl Med* 1994;8:159–162.

Lim-Dunham JE, Feinstein KA, Yousefzadeh DK, et al. Sonographic demonstration of a normal thyroid gland excludes ectopic thyroid in patients with thyroglossal duct cyst. *Am J Roentgenol* 1995;164:1489–1491.

McHenry CR, Danish R, Murphy T, et al. Atypical thyroglossal duct cyst: a rare cause for a solitary cold thyroid nodule in childhood. *Am Surg* 1993;59:223–228.

Urao M, Teitelbaum DH, Miyano T. Lingual thyroglossal duct cyst: a unique surgical approach. *J Pediatr Surg* 1996;31:1574–1576.

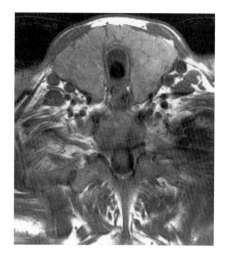 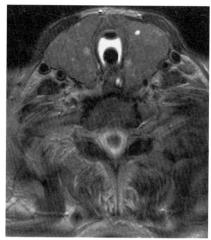

FIGURE 30.1A   **FIGURE 30.1B**

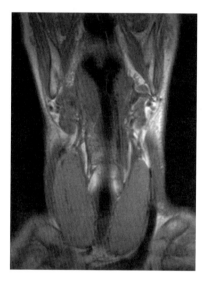

FIGURE 30.1C

CLINICAL HISTORY

A 52-year-old man with an anterior neck mass presented with recent onset of signs of thyrotoxicosis.

FINDINGS

Axial MRI of the neck shows an enlarged, homogeneous thyroid gland without invasion or narrowing of the airway (Fig. 30.1A). The margins of the gland are lobulated but well defined. On T2-weighted images, there are scattered areas of increased signal intensity (Fig. 30.1B). The coronal T1-weighted images show the cranial caudal extent of the gland (Fig. 30.1C). No cervical lymphadenopathy is noted.

DIAGNOSIS

Goiter due to Graves' disease

DISCUSSION

Seventy-five percent of patients with goiter present with a chronic asymptomatic anterior neck mass and seek medical attention for cosmetic reasons. Most commonly, goiters are detected by physicians during routine physical examination. A small percentage present with compressive symptoms, symptoms of thyroid dysfunction (either hypothyroidism or hyperthyroidism), or sudden growth associated with pain. Compressive symptoms include dyspnea, stridor, dysphagia, and hoarseness and are seen more often in patients with substernal or intrathoracic goiter.

Even though 80% of patients with goiter are euthyroid at presentation, subclinical hypothyroidism or hyperthyroidism may be present and therefore thyroid function tests should be performed in the initial evaluation. Sudden enlargement and pain are usually associated with hemorrhage into a follicular cyst but they may also signal malignant transformation. The clinical history should address not only the possible causes of goiter (e.g., recent viral infection, pregnancy or recent delivery, autoimmune disorders, or exposure to goitrogens) but also the risk of malignancy (e.g., rate of growth, family history of thyroid cancer, presence of multiple endocrine neoplasia syndromes).

The nationality and residence of each patient should be ascertained to rule out the possibility of iodine deficiency. On physical examination, the volume, mobility, and consistency of the gland, and the presence of any dominant nodules or cervical and supraclavicular lymphadenopathy should be evaluated. The volume of the gland should be recorded in the patient's clinical chart to allow for future comparison and determine the success of therapy. Auscultation of the thyroid gland may detect the presence of a bruit, indicating increased vascularity, typical of Graves' disease. Direct or indirect laryngoscopy should also be performed to evaluate vocal cord mobility. Examination of other major organs and systems (particularly the cardiovascular system, skin, and eyes) is important to determine the presence of clinical thyroid dysfunction. Biochemical analysis including determination of blood levels of thyroid-stimulating hormone (TSH), free T3 and T4, and antithyroid antibodies may be required. After an adequate history is obtained and physical examination and biochemical testing are performed, most patients do not require further diagnostic tests. When the goiter is multinodular at palpation, fine-needle aspiration (FNA) of any dominant or enlarging nodules is advised to exclude malignancy.

Goiter is a nonspecific term meaning diffuse enlargement of the thyroid gland, which may be seen in a large variety of pathologic processes affecting the thyroid gland. However, it is commonly used as a synonym for nontoxic or euthyroid goiter. *Endemic goiter,* defined as goiter in at least 10% of the pediatric population, is the most common cause of goiter worldwide. Seventy-five percent of cases occur in developing countries, which lack iodine prophylaxis, and the remainder occur in mountainous regions of Europe and Asia. In the United States, endemic goiter is virtually nonexistent and most cases of goiter are sporadic. The incidence of goiter in iodine-replete populations has been estimated at between 4% and 6%. Nonendemic goiter is more common in women and in the elderly.

The incidence of malignant degeneration varies from 1% to 4% and increases with age and prior exposure to radiation.

The pathophysiologic mechanism common to all causes of goiter is an excessive stimulation of the epithelial follicular cells leading either to excessive replication and formation of hyperplastic follicles or to hyperfunction with excessive production and accumulation of colloid material. In endemic goiter, the gland hypertrophies in an attempt to produce more thyroid hormone with less available iodine. Most goitrogens act through the hypothalamic-hypophyseal loop, producing an increase in TSH. Another common mechanism is the stimulation by thyroid antibodies that act directly on the TSH receptors in the follicular cells in Graves' disease or that damage the thyroid cells such as in Hashimoto's thyroiditis. Goiter may also result from congenital enzymatic deficiencies impairing iodine uptake or organification, or it may be part of congenital syndromes such as Pendred's syndrome (congenital deafness and goiter). Common goitrogens include iodine rich foods (soy beans, sea weeds), iodine-containing drugs (Pendred, contrast material, antiseptics), and drugs containing salts that compete with iodine for thyroid absorption (lithium). The typical progression of goiter is from diffuse enlargement of the thyroid gland to increasing nodularity.

Imaging of goiter has 5 major goals: (a) to provide an accurate assessment of glandular volume and morphology, (b) to evaluate compression of adjacent structures including the airway, (c) to determine the functional status of clinically suspicious nodules, (d) to detect imaging features suggestive of malignant degeneration, and (e) to direct FNA. However, the cost-effectiveness of imaging and the preferred modalities for addressing these problems are the subject of controversy. Surgical candidates should have a cross-sectional imaging study to determine the anatomy of the gland and its relationship to adjacent structures. MRI is preferred over CT because it does not involve ionizing radiation, does not require contrast administration, and allows for multiplanar evaluation.

MRI gives optimal delineation of the size and configuration of the gland. The coronal and sagittal images are particularly helpful in assessing the craniocaudal extent of the gland, detecting the presence of any mediastinal components (plunging goiter), and assessing the status of the airway and esophagus.

The use of iodine-based contrast materials on CT not only may precipitate a hyperthyroid crisis but also will interfere with subsequent scintigraphic studies, laboratory tests, and radioiodine therapy. The only advantage of CT is better sensitivity in detection of thyroid calcifications, which, although nonspecific, may be of diagnostic value. The use of scintigraphic studies to evaluate the functional status of thyroid nodules is questionable because fine needle aspiration biopsy (FNAB) is more accurate than scintigraphy in the assessment of thyroid nodules. Scintigraphic studies may be performed with ^{123}I or ^{99m}Tc. The former is used to evaluate glandular function and the latter is used to evaluate glandular morphology.

Ultrasound is the optimal imaging modality for evaluation of the thyroid gland; it is widely available, rapid, and inexpensive. It is also very accurate in distinguishing solid and cystic lesions and can provide guidance for FNAs of any suspicious nonpalpable lesions.

Therapy of goiter should be directed to its cause. Therefore, it may include dietary iodine supplements, elimination of goitrogens, and therapy with antiinflammatory drugs and antithyroid drugs. Most patients with euthyroid goiters can be managed conservatively with clinical monitoring of the volume of the gland. However, surgical treatment may be required for cosmesis, alleviation of compressive symptoms, or malignant degeneration. Decrease in glandular volume may be achieved with antithyroid drugs such as levothyroxin, radioiodine, or surgery. Ultrasound-guided ethanol ablation of hyperfunctioning thyroid nodules has also been used with high success rates.

SUGGESTED READINGS

Daniels GH. Thyroid nodules and nodular thyroids: a clinical overview. *Compr Ther* 1996;22:239–250.

Dworkin HJ, Meier DA, Kaplan M. Advances in the management of patients with thyroid disease. *Semin Nucl Med* 1995;25:205–220.

Hurley DL, Gharib H. Evaluation and management of multinodular goiter. *Otolaryngol Clin North Am* 1996;29:527–540.

Naik KS, Bury RF. Imaging the thyroid. *Clin Radiol* 1998;53:630–639.

Petrone LR. A primary care approach to the adult patient with nodular thyroid disease. *Arch Fam Med* 1996;5:92–100.

Singh B, Lucente FE, Shaha AR. Substernal goiter: a clinical review. *Am J Otolaryngol* 1994;15:409–416.

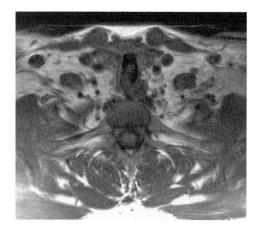

FIGURE 31.1A

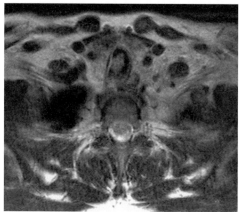

FIGURE 31.1B

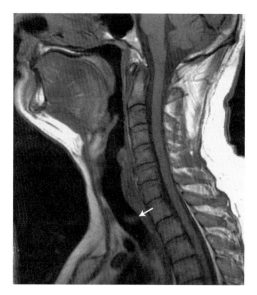

FIGURE 31.1C

CLINICAL HISTORY

The patient is a 35-year-old man with chronic cough. After clinical examination, an MR scan was requested to evaluate a possible mass.

FINDINGS

Axial T1-weighted MR images at the level of the upper trachea reveal a pedunculated posterolateral soft tissue mass, which extends into the airway (Fig. 31.1A). T2-weighted images show a similar appearance (Fig. 31.1B). There is no destruction of the trachea or invasion of surrounding structures. The airway is significantly narrowed. The sagittal image shows the location of the mass just inferior to the cricoid cartilage (Fig. 31.1C).

DIAGNOSIS

Primary tracheal squamous carcinoma.

DISCUSSION

The clinical manifestations of tracheal tumors are primarily through the effects of partial airway obstruction. Cough is present in half the patients and dyspnea and wheezing are common. Approximately 25% of the tracheal lumen must be occluded before obstructive symptoms become dominant. Hemoptysis is present in 10% of patients with benign tracheal tumors and in more than 50% of those with malignant tumors.

Primary neoplasms of the trachea are rare, especially compared with neoplasms of the larynx or lung. Depending on the series reported, there is approximately one carcinoma of the trachea for every 20 carcinomas of the larynx and one tracheal carcinoma for every 180 lung carcinomas. The reason for this remains unclear. Secondary involvement of the trachea by carcinomas is much more common with 10 to 20 cases for every case of primary tracheal carcinoma.

Primary tracheal tumors in the pediatric age group are distinctly uncommon, with 90% of tumors occurring in adults. In the pediatric population, less than 10% of tumors are malignant. In adults, 50% of primary tracheal neoplasms are malignant. Of these, most are carcinomas. Half of these carcinomas are the familiar squamous cell carcinoma. In patients with primary tracheal carcinoma, synchronous or metachronous tumors manifest in 20%. Benign nonneoplastic soft tissue masses such as granulomas may occur in the trachea but they do not tend to have an aggressive radiographic appearance.

The diagnosis is suggested by the presence of a mass narrowing the tracheal lumen. Secondary invasion by malignancies of adjacent structures may have a similar appearance and are much more common than primary tracheal carcinoma. With a benign appearing tracheal mass, other considerations such as granuloma or papilloma should be considered. When tracheal lumen narrowing is due to cartilage changes without a discrete mass, chondromalacia should be considered.

SUGGESTED READINGS

Holbert JM, Strollo DC. Imaging of the normal trachea. *J Thorac Imaging* 1995;10:171–179.
Weber AL. Radiologic evaluation of the trachea. *Chest Surg Clin North Am* 1996;6:637–673.

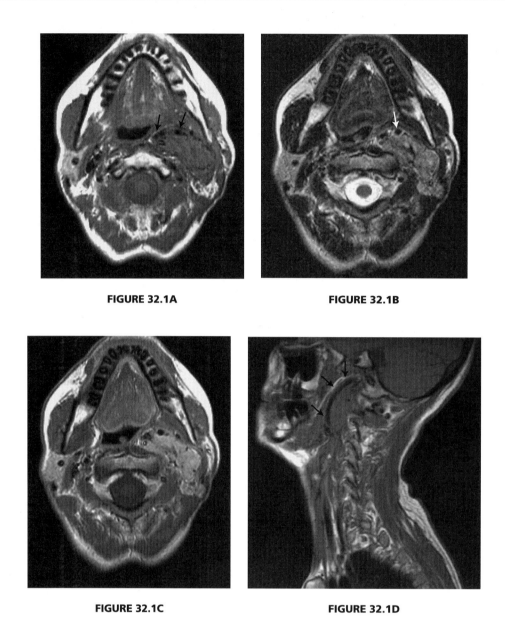

FIGURE 32.1A

FIGURE 32.1B

FIGURE 32.1C

FIGURE 32.1D

CLINICAL HISTORY

A 45-year-old female patient was referred for evaluation of a new parapharyngeal space mass.

FINDINGS

A mass is demonstrated on T1- and T2-weighted axial images (Fig. 32.1A, B). It is located in the post-styloid compartment of the left parapharyngeal space as evidenced by the anterior displacement of the carotid arteries. Numerous serpentine signal voids are noted within and around the mass, suggesting hypervascularity. Postcontrast, the mass demonstrates intense enhancement (Fig. 32.1C). The sagittal image shows that the lesion is well below the level of the jugular foramen (Fig. 32.1D).

DIAGNOSIS

Glomus vagale.

DISCUSSION

Paragangliomas are slowly growing neuroendocrine neoplasms that arise from neural crest derivatives. In the case of glomus vagale, this is usually from the nodose ganglion of the vagus nerve. Chemodectoma, glomus tumor, nonchromaffin paraganglioma, and neurocristopathic tumor are other names given to this lesion. Paragangliomas of the head and neck can be classified by their locations. Tumors of carotid and vagal locations are most frequent. Tympanic and jugular tumors are less frequent.

Precapillary arteriovenous shunts and nonchromaffin cells are characteristic of the histologic appearance of these tumors. Sheets of tumor cells are often divided into ball-like clusters ("Zelballen") separated by thin fibrovascular septa.

The most frequent presenting symptom is a mass in the cervical or pharyngeal area, and 30% of patients have cranial nerve impairment that frequently manifests by neck hypoesthesia and pharyngeal pain. A woman in her 40s with a painful pharyngeal mass associated with tenth and twelfth cranial nerve impairment has a very high likelihood of having a vagal paraganglioma. This tumor may arise from either intravagal and extravagal paraganglions. An intravagal tumor may produce rapid vagal impairment.

Paragangliomas and schwannomas are the two most common diagnoses for a post-styloid parapharyngeal space mass. Vagal paragangliomas represent approximately 10% of all branchial paragangliomas and show a female dominance of 2.5:1.

There is a tendency of multicentricity of tumors (10%), especially in a patient with a carotid body tumor showing familial tendency (26%). Vagal and carotid body tumors are more likely to be multifocal than paragangliomas in other head and neck locations. The incidence of true malignancy showing metastasis is less than 5%.

A vagal paraganglioma is easily delineated on CT and MR with its well-encapsulated and hypervascular nature. The mass effect on adjacent vessels is quite different from that of a carotid body tumor and may be a clue for differentiation. Conventional angiography is no longer routinely used for diagnosis but is valuable for preoperative embolization. Some investigators are beginning to use color Doppler ultrasound to help characterize these lesions. A glomus vagale is generally located more cephalad than a carotid body tumor, which is characteristically located at the carotid bifurcation. Unlike glomus jugulare tumors, which are located at the jugular bulb, glomus vagale tumors are more caudad.

Schwannomas may occur in a similar post-styloid parapharyngeal space location with similar displacement of the carotid vessels as a glomus vagale. However, they are often less vascular, and therefore are without the "salt and pepper" appearance of the paraganglioma.

Surgery is the primary treatment for these lesions, with radiation therapy used as an alternative for complex cases. Preoperative embolization to control bleeding is the rule.

SUGGESTED READINGS

Cole JM, Beiler D. Long-term results of treatment for glomus jugulare and glomus vagale tumors with radiotherapy. *Laryngoscope* 1994;104:1461–1465.

Jansen JC, Baatenburg de Jong RJ, Schipper J, van der Mey AG, van Gils AP. Color Doppler imaging of paragangliomas in the neck. *J Clin Ultrasound* 1997;25:481–485.

Leverstein H, Castelijns JA, Snow GB. The value of magnetic resonance imaging in the differential diagnosis of parapharyngeal space tumours. *Clin Otolaryngol* 1995;20:428–433.

Som PM, Sacher M, Stollman AL, et al. Common tumors of the parapharyngeal space: refined imaging diagnosis. *Radiology* 1988;169:81–85.

Zak FG, Lawson W. *The paraganglionic chemoreceptor system. Physiology, pathology, and clinical medicine.* New York: Springer-Verlag, 1982.

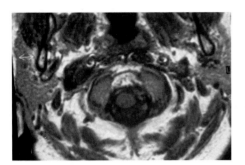 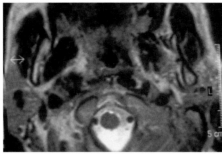 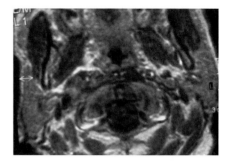

FIGURE 33.1A   FIGURE 33.1B   FIGURE 33.1C

CLINICAL HISTORY

A 68-year-old woman presents with hoarseness and dysphagia.

FINDINGS

There is a small mass in the post-styloid compartment of the right parapharyngeal space between the internal carotid artery and the jugular vein. The mass is hypointense on T1-weighted images (Fig. 33.1A) and heterogeneous on T2-weighted images (Fig. 33.1B), and enhances after gadolinium administration (Fig. 33.1C).

DIAGNOSIS

Vagus nerve schwannoma in the post-styloid compartment of the parapharyngeal space.

DISCUSSION

Twenty-five to forty-five percent of schwannomas occur in the head and neck. Schwannomas and neurofibromas are the most common nerve sheath tumors originating from the vagus nerve. Vagus nerve schwannomas account for 17% to 25% of all tumors in the parapharyngeal space. The peak incidence is between 30 and 60 years, but it can occur at any age.

The parapharyngeal space is a grossly rectangular space located deep to the masticator and parotid spaces and lateral to the mucosal pharyngeal space. In the suprahyoid neck, it is commonly divided by the styloid process into an anterior compartment (prestyloid), containing mostly fat and minor salivary glands, and a posterior compartment (post-styloid), also called the carotid space, containing the carotid artery, jugular vein, lymph nodes, cranial nerves IX through XI and the sympathetic chain. Most pathologic processes arising in the post-styloid compartment are lymphadenopathy, paragangliomas, or nerve sheath tumors. Cranial nerve X locates slightly posterior to and in between the carotid artery and the jugular vein. When a tumor arises from this nerve, the vascular structures of the carotid space tend to be displaced anteriorly and may also be splayed from each other.

Clinically, the patient may be asymptomatic with the lesion found incidentally on imaging studies. Those with symptoms may present with a slow-growing, painless neck mass, which may be fusiform, ovoid, or spherical, and which may be firm to rubbery hard on clinical examination. If the lesion is large enough, multiple dysfunctional vagal symptoms, such as hoarseness, dysphagia, dysphonia, as well as dyspnea, dysrhythmia, and symptoms related to sympathetic chain compression (Horner's syndrome), may be experienced.

Pathologically, schwannomas are well-encapsulated lesions, usually ovoid in shape with the long axis of the tumor following the course of the nerve. Vagal schwannomas usually arise near the nodosa ganglion, but they can be anywhere along the course of the vagal nerve. Multiple and bilateral lesions may occur in association with neurofibromatosis type II. Schwannomas originate from Schwann cells, made of two major tissue types: (a) Antoni A (compact Schwann cells with nuclear palisading), the cellular component, and (b) Antoni B (less dense cells arranged loosely), the myxoid component. When large, vagus nerve schwannoma can undergo cystic and hemorrhagic degeneration.

Other than location, the imaging features of vagus nerve schwannoma are nonspecific on both CT and MRI. On MRI, they are usually hypointense to isointense to muscle on T1-weighted images and slightly hyperintense on T2-weighted images. Depending on the presence of hemorrhage or cystic components, imaging features may vary. They are commonly hypovascular, but one third can be very vascular as a result of leakage of contrast into the extravascular space and they enhance intensely, making differentiation from paraganglioma difficult. However, the "salt and pepper" MR appearance and the arterial type of enhancement detected on dynamic CT studies, Doppler ultrasound, or conventional angiography are hallmarks of glomus tumors.

Other differential considerations include cervical sympathetic chain schwannoma and lymphoma. Lymphadenopathy are common lesions in the post-styloid compartment of the parapharyngeal space. Although they tend to be multiple and are associated with either inflammatory and infectious or neoplastic processes, they may be solitary and be the first sign of an occult malignancy. Complete surgical excision with sparing of the vagus nerve is the treatment of choice and is usually performed using a transcervical approach. Because recurrence or malignant degeneration is rare and vagus nerve damage is a possible sequela, several authors favor a conservative management for asymptomatic lesions.

SUGGESTED READINGS

Curtin H. Separation of the masticator space from the parapharyngeal space. *Radiology* 1987;163:195–204.

Furukawa M, et al. Differentiation between schwannoma of the vagus nerve and schwannoma of the cervical sympathetic chain by imaging diagnosis. *Laryngoscope* 1996;106:1548–1552.

Hamza A, et al. Neurilemomas of the parapharyngeal space. *Arch Otolaryngol Head Neck Surg* 1997;123:622–629.

Kempf HG, Becker G, Weber BP, et al. Diagnostic and clinical outcome of neurogenic tumors in the head and neck area. *J Otorhinolaryngol* 1995;57:273–278.

Leverstein H, Castelijns JA, Snow GB. The value of magnetic resonance imaging in the differential diagnosis of parapharyngeal space tumors. *Clin Otolaryngol* 1995;20:428–433.

Pensak ML, Gluckman JL, Shumrik KA. Parapharyngeal space tumors: an algorithm for evaluation and management. *Laryngoscope* 1994;104:1170–1173.

Som PM, Curtin HD. Lesions of the parapharyngeal space. Role of MR imaging. *Otolaryngol Clin North Am* 1995;28:515–542.

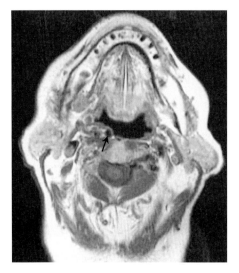

FIGURE 34.1A

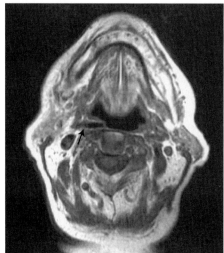

FIGURE 34.1B

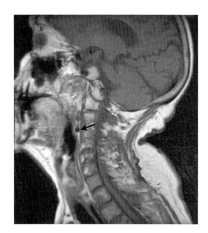

FIGURE 34.1C

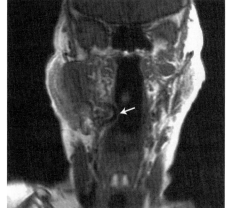

FIGURE 34.1D

CLINICAL HISTORY

An adult woman was brought to the clinic complaining of neck pain and sore throat. Physical examination demonstrated a nonpulsatile soft tissue fullness in the right posterior pharyngeal wall.

FINDINGS

Axial T1-weighted MR image through the mass shows a tubular signal void that represents the carotid artery (Fig. 34.1A, B). There is no evidence of associated mass. The T1-weighted coronal (Fig. 34.1C) and sagittal (Fig. 34.1D) images confirm that the mass is located at the carotid artery.

DIAGNOSIS

Medially deviated carotid artery.

DISCUSSION

The retropharyngeal space is a potential space that extends from the skull base to the level of the third thoracic vertebral body and and is bounded posteriorly by the prevertebral fascia and anteriorly by the retrovisceral fascia. Laterally, the ala fascia arises and crosses the retropharyngeal space from side to side, dividing it into an anterior and posterior portion. The retropharyngeal space primarily contains fat and lymph nodes. Several other spaces border the retropharyngeal space. The pharyngeal mucosal spaces of the nasopharynx, oropharynx, and hypopharynx are located anteriorly. The carotid space is located laterally. It contains the internal carotid artery, internal jugular vein, cranial nerves IX through XII, the cervical sympathetic plexus, and the external carotid artery branches.

Tortuous carotid arteries and congenital aberrant course of the carotid arteries are relatively uncommon problems of the retropharyngeal space. Awareness of these entities becomes significant when performing procedures such as oropharyngeal intubation, biopsy, abscess drainage, or other related surgeries because these could result in vascular injury with potentially disastrous results.

Less than 1% of the general population has congenital tortuosity of the internal carotid artery. This abnormal course results from failure of uncoiling of an embryologic bend present at the junction of the embryonic dorsal aorta and the third aortic arch. The aberrant vessel courses adjacent to the tonsillar capsule of the pharyngeal wall in close apposition with the superior constrictor muscle. Medial deviation of the carotid artery may also be seen with normal aging as an incidental finding. Redundancy of the carotid artery has also been related to a decrease in cerebral flow with rotational motion of the neck and stroke. This finding in older patients may sometimes be associated with vascular calcifications seen on lateral and frontal cervical radiographs. Calcified carotid arteries in normal position overlie the vertebrae on the lateral radiograph and can be seen lateral to the vertebrae on the frontal views. In patients with medial deviation of the carotid arteries, the calcified vessels are anterior to the vertebrae on the lateral view and are usually not visible or superimposed upon the vertebrae on the frontal view. CT or MR imaging with or without intravenous contrast enhancement is valuable for proper localization of the medial position of the carotid artery.

SUGGESTED READINGS

Cheung YK, Sham JST, Chan FL, et al. Computed tomography of the paranasopharyngeal spaces: normal variations and criteria for tumor extension. *Clin Radiol* 1992;45:109–113.

Colletti PM, Terk MR, Zee CS. Magnetic resonance angiography in the neck masses. *Comput Med Imaging Graph* 1996;20:379–388.

Davis WL, Harnsberger HR, Smoker WRK, et al. Retropharyngeal space: evaluation of normal anatomy and diseases with CT and MR imaging. *Radiology* 1990;174:59–64.

Poe LB, Manzione JV, Wasenko JJ, et al. Acute internal jugular vein thrombosis associated with pseudoabscess of the retropharyngeal space. *AJNR Am J Neuroradiol* 1995;16:892–896.

Schumacher WA, Schafig A, Kehrl W, et al. Variations in the course of the internal carotid artery: possible risks in the so-called standard operations in the area of the pharynx. *Laryngorhinootologie* 1998;77:517–520.

Silver AJ, Mawad ME, Hilal SK, et al. Computed tomography of the carotid space and related cervical spaces. *Radiology* 1984;150:723–728.

Som PM, Biller HF, Lawson W, et al. Parapharyngeal space masses: an updated protocol based upon 104 cases. *Radiology* 1984;153:149–156.

CASE 35

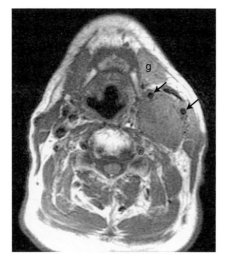

FIGURE 35.1A

FIGURE 35.1B

FIGURE 35.1C

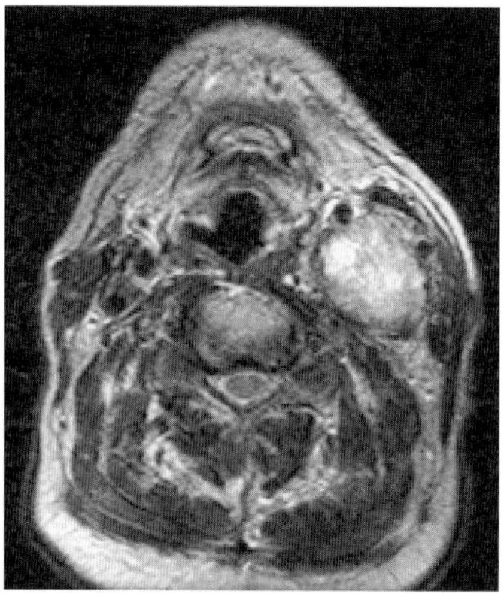

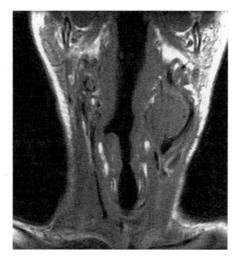

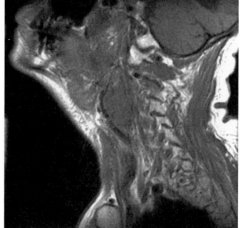

FIGURE 35.1D

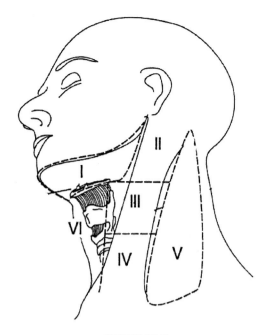

FIGURE 35.2

CLINICAL HISTORY

A middle-aged man presents with a new neck mass on the left.

FINDINGS

Axial T1-weighted MR image shows a large mass posterior to the submandibular gland. The carotid arteries are splayed and displaced anteriorly (Fig. 35.1A). On T2-weighted images, the central portion shows scattered areas of increased signal intensity, suggesting necrosis (Fig. 35.1B). The coronal image shows the mass and no evidence of other pathology (Fig. 35.1C). The sagittal scan again shows anterior displacement of the vessels (Fig. 35.1D).

DIAGNOSIS

Necrotic lymph node from squamous cell carcinoma metastases. No primary tumor was identified.

DISCUSSION

Squamous cell carcinoma is the most common malignant neoplasm of the upper aerodigestive tract. One of the most important factors that influence therapeutic outcome of patients with this disease is the presence of cervical lymph node metastases. A single nodal metastasis reduces the patient's survival rate by approximately 50%, regardless of location or size of the primary tumor in the head and neck.

The descriptive nomenclature of cervical nodes has evolved through several different nodal classification systems. Cervical nodes were initially categorized by Rouviere into one of 10 principal groups based on their precise anatomic location. This was later slightly modified by the Union International Contre le Cancer (International Union Against Cancer [UICC]). Currently, an improved, simplified classification aims to eliminate misinterpretation caused by variation in terminology of cervical nodes as well as to provide standardization by using a level system. It is endorsed by the American Joint Committee on Cancer (AJCC) and the American Academy of Otolaryngology—Head and Neck Surgery (AAOHNS). Major cervical nodal groups are classified as level I through level VI (Fig. 35.2).

This classification is useful for understanding recent applications of conservative or selective neck dissection, in which a part of the cervical nodal groups are removed. Some nodal groups, such as retropharyngeal nodes and intraparotid nodes, are not included in this numeric classification and must still be referred to by their anatomic classification.

Before the development of CT, assessment of cervical nodal metastases was based completely on palpation of lymph nodes as detected by physical examination. The inaccuracy of the physical examination has been documented in a number of studies. False-negative and false-positive rates of the physical examination are 15% to 20% and 30% to 50%, respectively. CT and MRI have improved the accuracy of nodal staging over physical examination. Both techniques allow visualization of nonpalpable nodes deep to the sternocleidomastoid muscle or in the retropharyngeal space.

Clinically occult, normal-sized nodes with central necrosis or with extracapsular spread can be identified as metastases by CT or MR. Borderline-sized nodes without necrosis or extracapsular spread remain indeterminate by both CT or MR. Size has been a widely used criterion to determine the presence of nodal metastases. Because size data are a continuum, the relative sensitivity and specificity of any size criteria can be adjusted by changes in the threshold dimensions, depending on a clinical setting. Small metastatic nodes can be missed. Conversely, large reactive nodes cannot be differentiated consistently from metastatic nodes.

In the early era of CT, size criteria for nodal metastases were established by investigating the range of normal variation in size of lymph nodes in subjects without cancer. The initial criterion was that "discrete lymph nodes larger than 1.5 cm are considered metastases." More recently, size criteria have been reassessed with extensive pathologic analysis.

One study suggested that a minimum (short) axial diameter of 11 mm for the jugulodigastric nodes and 10 mm for all other nodes more accurately reflects the presence of metastases. Another multicenter study analyzing nodal size in 100 neck dissections revealed that 46% of pathologic nodes were less than 1 cm and 22% of pathologic nodes were between 1 and 1.5 cm in diameter. Thus, a significant number of metastatic nodes are missed (false negative) by simple size criteria.

In patients with squamous cell carcinoma, central nodal low attenuation with ring enhancement is likely to represent the presence of necrosis or tumor itself within metastatic nodes. However, a homogeneous appearance of lymph nodes on CT or MRI does not exclude the presence of nodal metastasis. Normal fat deposition, as well as abscess formation in patients with infectious disease, may mimic central necrosis of lymph nodes.

Spread of the malignancy beyond the lymph node "capsule" has a strong negative impact on patient prognosis. One study reported that the presence of extracapsular spread reduces the 2-year survival rate of patients by approximately 50%. Indeed, when extracapsular spread is pathologically evident, postoperative radiation therapy is mandatory. CT and MR findings indicative of extracapsular spread include irregular nodal boundaries and obliteration of the adjacent fat planes if there has been no recent infection, radiation therapy, or surgical intervention in this region. All of these processes cause irregular nodal borders and obliteration of fat planes.

A variety of cervical nodal dissection procedures have been developed for treatment of nodal metastases in head and neck cancer. Radical neck dissection (RND) involves en bloc removal of all lymph nodes from level I through level V along with the sternocleidomastoid muscle, internal jugular vein, and spinal accessory nerve. Significant morbidity is associated with RND, such as shoulder dropping and pain. The idea of a less invasive neck dissection has been developed to minimize functional and cosmetic deficits while maintaining adequate disease control. As more conservative neck dissections have become available without sacrificing prognosis, more accurate and tissue-specific presurgical imaging studies are necessary. Radiation therapy is added in selected cases.

SUGGESTED READINGS

Anzai Y, Brunberg JA, Lufkin R. Imaging of nodal metastases in the head and neck. *J MRI* 1997;7:774–783.

Don D, Anzai Y, Lufkin RB, et al. Evaluation of cervical lymph node metastases in squamous cell carcinoma of the head and neck. *Laryngoscope* 1995;105:669–674.

Som PM. Detection of metastases in cervical lymph nodes; CT and MR criteria and differential diagnosis. *AJR Am J Roentgenol* 1992;158:961–969.

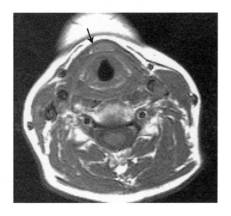

FIGURE 36.1A

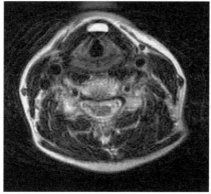

FIGURE 36.1B

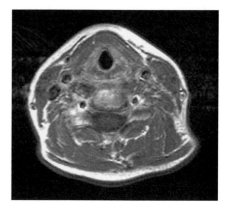

FIGURE 36.1C

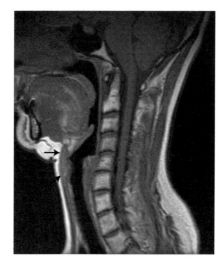

FIGURE 36.1D

CLINICAL HISTORY

Incidental mass detected on MR scan for other indications.

FINDINGS

Axial MR scans show a small rounded mass in the midline (Fig. 36.1A). On T2-weighted images, it appears to be cystic and have thin walls (Fig. 36.1B). On postcontrast views, it does not enhance (Fig. 36.1C). The sagittal view shows that it extends from the hyoid bone inferiorly toward the thyroid gland (Fig. 36.1D).

DIAGNOSIS

Thyroglossal duct cyst.

DISCUSSION

The thyroglossal duct is an epithelial lined tubular structure extending from the foramen cecum, around the inferior border of the hyoid bone to the pyramidal lobe of the thyroid bed. It is formed by the third week of gestation and normally involutes by the tenth. If any portion fails to involute, the secretory epithelial lining may cause a cyst to be formed. Although these are congenital lesions, they often do not present until there is inflammation or blockage of drainage. For a more complete discussion of these lesions, please see the other case of thyroglossal duct cyst (Case 29).

SUGGESTED READINGS

Kawanaka M, Sugimoto Y, Suehiro M, et al. Thyroid imaging in a typical case of acute suppurative thyroiditis with abscess formation due to infection from a persistent thyroglossal duct. *Ann Nucl Med* 1994;8:159–162.

Lim-Dunham JE, Feinstein KA, Yousefzadeh DK, et al. Sonographic demonstration of a normal thyroid gland excludes ectopic thyroid in patients with thyroglossal duct cyst. *AJR Am J Roentgenol* 1995;164:1489–1491.

McHenry CR, Danish R, Murphy T, et al. Atypical thyroglossal duct cyst: a rare cause for a solitary cold thyroid nodule in childhood. *Am Surg* 1993;59:223–228.

Urao M, Teitelbaum DH, Miyano T. Lingual thyroglossal duct cyst: a unique surgical approach. *J Pediatr Surg* 1996;31:1574–1576.

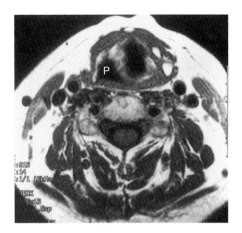

FIGURE 37.1A

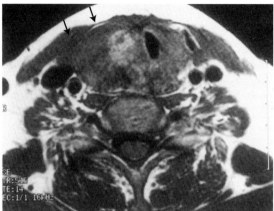

FIGURE 37.1B

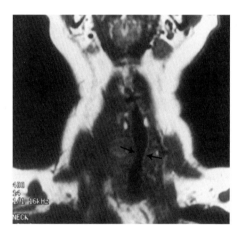

FIGURE 37.1C

CLINICAL HISTORY

A 58-year-old woman presents with a rapidly enlarging neck mass, progressive hoarseness, inspiratory dyspnea, and dysphagia. On physical examination a hard woody mass is palpated in the right lateral and anterior neck, fixed to the surrounding structures. On laryngoscopy, right vocal cord paralysis is noted.

FINDINGS

Axial T1-weighted MR image of the neck showing enlargement of the right pyriform sinus resulting from anteromedial deviation of the aryepiglottic fold (Fig. 37.1A). Lower axial T1-weighted images show an asymmetric thyroid gland resulting from enlargement of the right thyroid lobe. In addition, this lobe has two ill-defined nodular regions—one medial, adjacent to the trachea, and the other in the retrotracheal space. The largest nodule is hyperintense, possibly representing a nodular goiter with high protein content or hemorrhage. The remainder of this right lobe is markedly hypointense when compared with the contralateral side, and its margins are ill defined. There is obscuration of the fascial planes of the right sternocleidomastoid muscle, strap muscles, anterior aspect of the right internal jugular vein, and prevertebral muscles. The retrotracheal component occupies the tracheoesophageal groove and blends with the proximal esophagus, which is not clearly identified. The trachea is displaced anteriorly and to the left, and is narrowed in its transverse diameter (Fig. 37.1B). Coronal T1-weighted image shows the craniocaudal extent of the lesion and tracheal stenosis, with a 50% reduction in transverse tracheal caliber (Fig. 37.1C).

DIAGNOSIS

Riedel's thyroiditis with right vocal cord paralysis.

DISCUSSION

Thyroiditis is a general term used to designate a variety of inflammatory conditions occurring in the thyroid gland. They are classified according to their clinical presentation into acute, subacute, and chronic forms, and further subclassified according to etiology or pathology. The acute form is usually associated with an infectious process caused by bacterial or fungal agents and is also referred to as acute suppurative thyroiditis. The subacute category comprises two different conditions: subacute granulomatous thyroiditis (Quervain's thyroiditis), which is thought to result from a viral infection, and subacute lymphocytic thyroiditis, which likely represents an autoimmune entity differing from Hashimoto's thyroiditis in that it is self-limited and does not tend to cause irreversible hypothyroidism. This entity may be seen in the postpartum period and tends to recur in subsequent pregnancies. Chronic thyroiditis includes Hashimoto's thyroiditis (chronic lymphocytic thyroiditis), an autoimmune process that usually results in irreversible hypothyroidism, and Riedel's thyroiditis (invasive fibrous thyroiditis).

Except for acute suppurative thyroiditis, all other forms of thyroiditis are limited to the thyroid gland and do not commonly cause vocal cord paralysis, although they can cause compressive symptoms because of gland enlargement. The main clinical and imaging diagnostic mimic of Riedel's thyroiditis is anaplastic thyroid carcinoma, which may present in the same age group and with an indistinguishable clinico-radiologic picture. Thyroid lymphoma with a florid reactive desmoplastic reaction and the fibrosing variant of Hashimoto's thyroiditis may also be very difficult to distinguish from Riedel's thyroiditis pathologically. However, thyroid lymphoma does not tend to have a hard consistency on palpation and Hashimoto's thyroiditis, even the sclerosing variant, does not cross the boundaries of the thyroid gland.

Patients with Riedel's thyroiditis typically present with a rapidly enlarging neck mass, causing compressive symptoms such as hoarseness, inspiratory dyspnea, stridor, and dysphagia. Hoarseness may result from direct laryngeal extension, but more commonly results from involvement of the recurrent laryngeal nerve in the tracheoesophageal groove. Mediastinal extent may occur and be responsible for venous hypertensive syndromes such as superior vena cava syndrome. The disease may first appear in an otherwise normal gland or a preexisting goiter. Rarely, the gland may be normal in size and show a single nodular lesion. Symptoms and signs of hypothyroidism should be sought, although these tend to appear in the later phases when there has been extensive replacement of the thyroid gland parenchyma by fibrotic tissue.

It is important to ask about symptoms related to other fibrosclerotic processes, such as renal problems, hypertension, visual deficits, or jaundice. Euthyroidism or hypothyroidism is the rule and positivity for antithyroid antibodies is present in as many as 67% of cases.

Further diagnostic tests should include imaging studies and fine-needle aspiration (FNA) or surgical biopsy to make a definitive diagnosis and, especially, to exclude malignancy.

Riedel's thyroiditis is best described as a benign fibrotic process with aggressive features, partially or completely involving the thyroid gland and extending beyond the confines of the gland into the soft tissues of the neck. Since first described, multiple terms have been used to refer to this entity, including Riedel's struma, struma thyroiditis, and invasive fibrosing thyroiditis.

It is a rare condition, with an estimated incidence of 0.05% determined in the largest series of thyroid resections reported to date. The female-to-male ratio varies between 3:1 and 5:1, and the age group most commonly affected is between the fourth and seventh decades, with a peak incidence in the late forties. The disease may be unilateral or bilateral. There is a well-known association with other fibrosclerosing diseases including retroperitoneal and mediastinal fibrosis, orbital pseudotumor (sclerosing variety), and Addison's disease.

The etiology of Riedel's thyroiditis is unknown. There are two main theories, one suggesting an autoimmune process, which may be the same or different from the one responsible for Hashimoto's thyroiditis, and the other suggesting a localized or systemic fibrosclerosing inflammatory process.

FNA results are often nondiagnostic because of the increased consistency and hypocellularity of the gland. They may also be misleading with a few described cases of false-positive findings for carcinoma. Surgical biopsy is usually required for accurate diagnosis.

Imaging studies, besides providing useful diagnostic information, are required to determine the extent of disease and to exclude other sites of systemic involvement. Cross-sectional imaging of the orbits, mediastinum, or abdomen may be required in selected cases.

MRI, because of its multiplanar capability, adequately depicts the extent of the lesion and does not necessitate intravenous contrast. The gland may be partially or diffusely enlarged and the involved portions tend to be hypointense on both T1-weighted and T2-weighted images. These are the signal characteristics of fibrotic tissue, although amyloid deposits and hemochromatosis may share these same features on MRI. MRI may allow distinction from Hashimoto's thyroiditis, which tends to be markedly hyperintense on T2-weighted images. Less commonly, the gland is heterogeneous in signal intensity, especially when the disease is superimposed upon a preexisting goiter. Extracapsular extension manifests as irregularity of the margins of the gland, obscuration of the fascial planes, and obvious invasion of the surrounding structures. When the isthmus of the gland is involved, infiltration of the strap muscles and skin may be seen. Other structures frequently invaded include the sternocleidomastoid muscle, carotid space, tracheo-esophageal groove, and postcricoid and retropharyngeal regions. Airway deviation and stenosis is a frequent finding, as is indistinctness of the esophagus. The presence of cervical lymphadenopathy favors malignancy, most likely anaplastic thyroid carcinoma. Because recurrence is seen in a high percentage of cases, imaging follow-up is usually required.

Surgery may be required to alleviate compressive symptoms and for cosmetic reasons, or to make the definitive diagnosis when the FNA is nondiagnostic or doubtful. Tracheostomy may be required for life-threatening airway compromise, including cases of bilateral vocal cord paralysis. When malignancy is excluded, surgery should be limited to avoid complications resulting from attempted dissection of the invasive fibrotic tissue from surrounding structures.

The use of tamoxifen in fibrogenic disorders is being extensively evaluated and has had differing success rates. Radiation has no role in treatment of this disorder.

SUGGESTED READINGS

Bagnasco M, Passalacqua G, Pronzato C, et al. Fibrous invasive (Riedel's) thyroiditis with critical response to steroid treatment. *J Endocrinol Invest* 1995;18:305–307.

Brady OH, Hehir DJ, Heffernan SJ. Riedel's thyroiditis—case report and literature review. *Ir J Med Sci* 1994;163:176–177.

Elewaut D, Rubens R, Elewaut A, et al. Lusoria dysphagia in a patient with retroperitoneal fibrosis and Riedel's thyroiditis. *J Intern Med* 1996;239:75–78.

Few J, Thompson NW, Angelos P, et al. Riedel's thyroiditis: treatment with tamoxifen. *Surgery* 1996;120:993–998; discussion 998–999.

Heufelder AE, Goellner JR, Bahn RS, et al. Tissue eosinophilia and eosinophil degranulation in Riedel's invasive fibrous thyroiditis. *J Clin Endocrinol Metab* 1996;81:977–984.

Heufelder AE, Hay ID. Further evidence for autoimmune mechanisms in the pathogenesis of Riedel's invasive fibrous thyroiditis [letter; comment]. *J Intern Med* 1995;238:85–86.

Intenzo CM, Park CH, Kim SM, et al. Clinical, laboratory, and scintigraphic manifestations of subacute and chronic thyroiditis. *Clin Nucl Med* 1993;18:302–306.

Julie C, Vieillefond A, Desligneres S, et al. Hashimoto's thyroiditis associated with Riedel's thyroiditis and retroperitoneal fibrosis. *Pathol Res Pract* 1997;193:573–577; discussion 578.

Wan SK, Chan JK, Tang SK. Paucicellular variant of anaplastic thyroid carcinoma. A mimic of Reidel's thyroiditis. *Am J Clin Pathol* 1996;105:388–393.

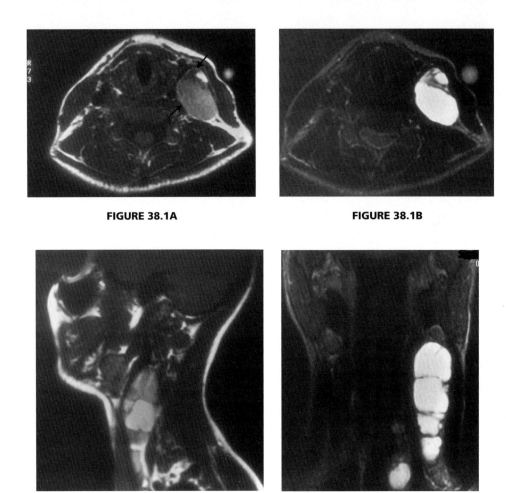

FIGURE 38.1A

FIGURE 38.1B

FIGURE 38.1C

FIGURE 38.1D

CLINICAL HISTORY

A young woman presents with a painless lower neck mass.

FINDINGS

Axial T1-weighted images show a heterogeneous mass deep to the sternocleidomastoid muscle (Fig. 38.1A). Sagittal T1-weighted images show its lobulated appearance with multiple thin-walled compartments of varying signal intensity (Fig. 38.1C). Axial and coronal T2-weighted images show striking high signal consistent with a high fluid content (Fig. 38.1B, D).

DIAGNOSIS

Lymphangioma.

DISCUSSION

Lymphangiomas are benign malformations of the lymphatic system. Most lymphangiomas occur during childhood, with 60% present at birth and 80% presenting by 2 years of age. This corresponds to the period when the greatest development of the lymphatic system occurs. There is no sex predominance. Some adult lymphangiomas may be of traumatic rather than developmental origin. Lymphangiomas are generally painless compressible neck masses. Airway obstruction is not uncommon in children. Cystic hygromas classically occur in the posterior triangle but may extend more anteriorly.

Lymphangiomas are nonencapsulated lesions of lymphoid tissue. Most authors believe they are malformations rather than true neoplasms. They are classified into three groups, based on the size of the lymphatic spaces within the mass: (a) lymphangioma simplex masses are composed of thin-walled capillary-sized channels, (b) cavernous lymphangiomas have more dilated lymphatics with fibrous adventitia, and (c) cystic hygromas have large cysts up to several centimeters in diameter. The radiographic appearance of these types overlap. In fact, all three tissue types may occur in the same lesion.

Ultrasound is valuable in imaging these lesions, especially in the perinatal period. CT and MRI are useful for defining the full extent of the lesions. Accurate delineation of lesion extension is important for preoperative diagnosis, surgical planning, and assessing recurrence.

Lymphangiomas are characteristically soft and conform to existing tissue spaces rather than distorting surrounding structures. Because of their large cystic spaces, they do not typically enhance with contrast. They are low signal on T1-weighted images and high signal on T2-weighted images. Figure 2 shows the MR appearance on axial T1-weighted image (Fig. 38.2A) and on T2-weighted image (Fig. 38.2B, C). With infection or hemorrhage, these signal characteristics may change.

Surgery is the therapy of choice for most patients with this condition. Imaging is especially valuable in defining the full extent of the lesion to allow for a complete excision at surgery.

SUGGESTED READINGS

Borecky N, Gudinchet F, Laurini R, et al. Imaging of cervico-thoracic lymphangiomas in children. *Pediatr Radiol* 1995;25:127–130.

Dubois J, Garel L, Grignon A, et al. Imaging of hemangiomas and vascular malformations in children. *Acad Radiol* 1998;5:390–400.

Fung K, Poenaru D, Soboleski DA, et al. Impact of magnetic resonance imaging on the surgical management of cystic hygromas. *J Pediatr Surg* 1998;33:839–841.

Vazquez E, Enriquez G, Castellote A, et al. US, CT, and MR imaging of neck lesions in children. *Radiographics* 1995;15:105–122.

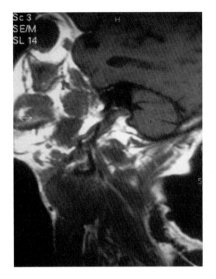

FIGURE 39.1A

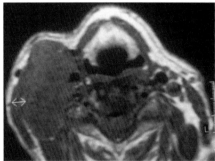

FIGURE 39.1B

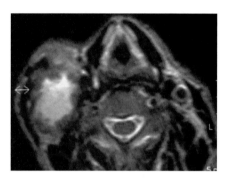

FIGURE 39.1C

CLINICAL HISTORY

A 65-year-old man who has previously undergone hemipelviglossectomy for squamous cell carcinoma of the oral tongue presents with a painful mass in the right lateral neck.

FINDINGS

Sagittal T1-weighted and axial T1- and T2-weighted images through the neck (Fig. 39.1A–C) show a large, heterogeneous, ill-defined mass in the right lateral neck encasing the right internal carotid artery. The carotid lumen is decreased when compared with the contralateral side but shows a flow void consistent with patency. The mass infiltrates the adjacent soft tissues, including the sternocleidomastoid muscle and subcutaneous fat, and shows large areas of necrosis.

DIAGNOSIS

Metastatic nodal mass with necrosis, extracapsular extension, and carotid artery encasement.

DISCUSSION

The presence of nodal metastases is one of the most important prognostic factors in patients with squamous cell carcinoma of the head and neck. A single nodal metastasis reduces survival rate by 50% regardless of location or "T" staging of the primary tumor. In addition, the presence of nodal necrosis, extracapsular extension, and vascular invasion further aggravates patient's outcome.

Prior to cross-sectional imaging, assessment of cervical node metastases relied solely on physical examination. However, neck palpation has a number of limitations: deep-seated, nonpalpable lymph nodes and normal-sized metastatic nodes are not amenable to clinical detection. Imaging, including ultrasound, CT, MRI, and, more recently, single photon emission computed tomography and positron emission tomography, overcome several of these limitations.

Imaging criteria for nodal metastases are based on number, size, distribution, and morphology of lymph nodes, architectural nodal changes, and their relationship to adjacent structures. Several size criteria have been used with values that vary according to node location. These include the longest and shortest lymph node axis and a relationship between those two. Because there is a wide variation in the size of both normal and metastatic lymph nodes, a wide overlap between normal and metastatic nodes is seen. Therefore, the sensitivity and specificity of size criteria depend on the threshold that is used in each clinical setting.

Architectural nodal changes result from infiltration of the medulla by neoplastic cells, which leads to loss of the normal nodal shape, loss of the fatty hilum, and a heterogeneous, ringlike pattern of enhancement typical for metastatic nodes. Central necrosis and ill-defined, infiltrative margins are also hallmarks of lymphadenopathy. However, these features are nonspecific and may be seen in several infectious and inflammatory conditions (e.g., tuberculous adenitis, cervical abscess, infected second branchial cleft cyst).

Extracapsular spread manifests as irregular nodal boundaries and obliteration of the adjacent fat planes. This may lead to vascular invasion with important therapeutic impact. Indirect signs of vascular invasion in order of increasing specificity include loss of fat planes between the nodal mass and the vessel, vessel encasement, and reduction or obliteration of the vascular lumen. MR angiography and conventional angiography may be useful in determining vessel patency and in detecting the irregularities of the vascular wall that are pathognomonic of vascular invasion.

Nodal metastases with carotid invasion are managed with radiation therapy with or without associated chemotherapy. Surgical options imply sacrifice of the internal carotid artery or a vascular bypass.

SUGGESTED READINGS

Anzai Y, Brunberg JA, Lufkin R. Imaging of nodal metastasis in the head and neck. *J Magn Reson Imaging* 1997;7:774–783.

Don D, Anzai Y, Fu YS, et al. Evaluation of cervical lymph node metastases in squamous cell carcinoma of the head and neck. *Laryngoscope* 1995;105:669–674.

Myers LL. Positron emission tomography in the evaluation of the negative neck in patients with oral cavity cancer. *J Otolaryngol* 1998;27:342–347.

Som PM. Detection of metastasis in cervical lymph nodes; CT and MR criteria and differential diagnosis. *Am J Roentgenol* 1992;158:961–969.

Wide JM. Magnetic resonance imaging in the assessment of cervical nodal metastasis in oral squamous cell carcinoma. *Clin Radiol* 1999;54:90.

Yusa H. Ultrasonographic criteria for diagnosis of cervical lymph node metastasis of squamous cell carcinoma in the oral and maxillofacial region. *J Oral Maxillofac Surg* 1999;57:41–48.

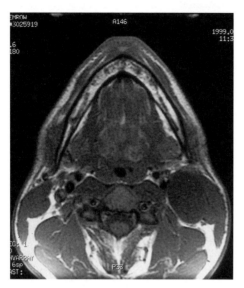

FIGURE 40.1

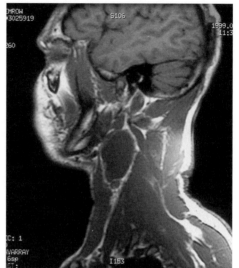

FIGURE 40.2

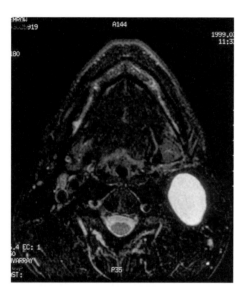

FIGURE 40.3

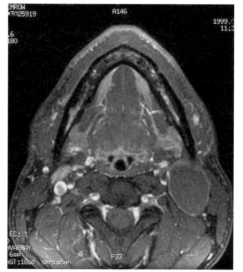

FIGURE 40.4

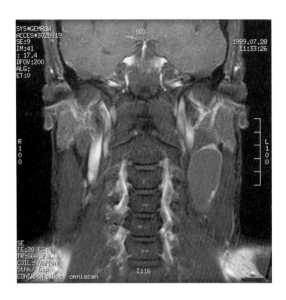

FIGURE 40.5

CLINICAL HISTORY

A 29-year-old man presents with a recurrent left neck mass after undergoing prior incision and drainage.

FINDINGS

Axial and sagittal T1-weighted images show a well-defined, homogeneously hypointense mass superficial to the left carotid artery and internal jugular vein, medial and slightly anterior to the proximal half of the left sternocleidomastoid muscle (Figs. 40.1, 40.2). The mass is isointense to slightly hyperintense to the CSF on the T2-weighted image (Fig. 40.3). Postcontrast axial and coronal T1-weighted images demonstrate mild rim enhancement.

DIAGNOSIS

Second branchial cleft cyst.

DISCUSSION

Branchial cleft cysts represent an incomplete proliferation, migration, or obliteration of one of the four branchial clefts. Second branchial cleft cysts are most common, accounting for more than 90%. They usually are centered in the anterior triangle at the mid-neck level and cross the common carotid artery bifurcation to end at the palatine tonsil.

The first branchial cleft cysts represent approximately 8% of all branchial cleft cysts. The lesions occur in the vicinity of the external auditory canal and may drain into it. Another location may be in the anterior triangle of the neck just inferior to the mandible.

The third branchial cleft cysts are uncommon, and are located anterior to the sternocleidomastoid muscle in the lower neck. The fourth branchial cleft cysts are very rare.

Clinically, most second branchial cleft cyst patients present with a smooth, nontender, fluctuant mass along the upper third of the sternocleidomastoid muscle. When not in communication with the external fistula, the cyst may go unnoticed until the second to fourth decades of life.

On CT, an uncomplicated branchial cleft cyst is homogeneously low in attenuation. However, a previously infected cyst, or one that has bled into its content, usually has cyst fluid that is denser than the normal mucoid density. A few thin septations may be noted either before or after needle aspiration.

On MRI, cyst contents usually have low T1-weighted and high T2-weighted signal intensity. However, often the cyst fluid may be sufficiently proteinaceous to be high signal intensity on both T1- and T2-weighted images. After contrast, the cyst wall (and not the fluid contents) enhance.

Branchial cleft cysts are treated by surgical resection with a low overall recurrence rate.

See also the other case in this volume for additional discussion of this entity and suggested readings (Case 25).

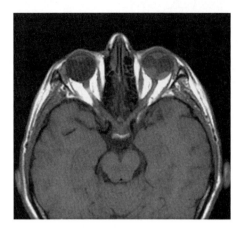

FIGURE 41.1A

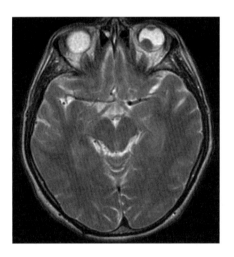

FIGURE 41.1B

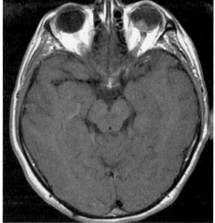

FIGURE 41.1C

CLINICAL HISTORY

A 60-year-old man notes a 2-week history of decreased vision in his left eye. Ophthalmic examination reveals a left choroidal mass.

FINDINGS

There is a lobulated choroidal mass on the left as seen on this axial T1-weighted image (Fig. 41.1A). On the T2-weighted images, there is a central mass with an adjacent subretinal fluid collection (Fig. 41.1B). The lesion is hyperintense (arrowhead) on postcontrast T1-weighted images after contrast (Fig. 41.1C). The contralateral globe is unremarkable.

DIAGNOSIS

Choroidal (uveal) melanoma.

DISCUSSION

Uveal melanoma is the most common primary ocular neoplasm in adults. It has an annual reported incidence of seven cases per million. There is no sexual predilection, although they are more common in individuals with light skin coloring. They are almost always unilateral.

Diagnosis is usually accomplished using standard ophthalmologic examination of ophthalmoscopy, sonography, or flourescein angiography. CT and more often MRI is valuable to evaluate extracapsular extension, which may occur in 10% to 15% of patients and may be difficult or impossible to evaluate with the prior techniques. Also in patients with "opaque media" (i.e., cataract, vitreous hemorrhage), direct ophthalmologic visualization may be impossible.

The tumor arises from malignant transformation of melanocytes in the uveal tract. The uveal tract is made up of the ciliary body, iris, and choroid. Melanoma in the ciliary body and choroid are believed to originate from preexisting nevi. Choroidal nevi are congenital lesions, usually detected late in the first decade of life and most commonly located in the posterior third of the choroid. They are usually not visible with high-resolution CT or MRI techniques.

The CT and MR appearance of choroidal melanoma is that of an enhancing choroidal mass. Initially, there is a smooth contour as the mass elevates Bruch's membrane (lamina vitrea). With more growth and rupture of the membrane, the tumor assumes a more characteristic mushroom shape. The adjacent retina commonly becomes elevated (detached) on either side of the tumor, leading to formation of subretinal fluid collections. These fluid collections can usually be differentiated from the primary mass on T2-weighted MR images. The imaging appearance of the melanoma may be mimicked by retinoblastoma, choroidal metastases, hemangioma, or intrachoroidal hemorrhage.

Using signal characteristics alone, choroidal hemorrhage may be mistaken for malignant uveal melanoma on clinical examination as well as on various imaging techniques. On MRI, acute choroidal hemorrhage appears as a moderately hypointense image on T2-weighted MR scans. Subacute choroidal hemorrhage may be seen as an area of heterogeneous signal intensity on both T1- and T2-weighted MR images. Chronic choroidal hemorrhage appears as hyperintense areas in both T1- and T2-weighted MR scans. Uveal metastases may be very difficult to differentiate from uveal melanoma. Most metastases, however, often appear hyperintense on T2-weighted MR images. Metastases from primary mucin-producing carcinoma and breast carcinoma may be very difficult to differentiate from uveal melanomas, because as melanomas, they may show hypointensity on T2-weighted images.

Although T1 and T2 shortening is seen in the majority of MR studies of patients with melanoma, the finding is not entirely sensitive or specific in the diagnosis of melanoma, because a small percentage of melanomas contain small amounts of melanin (amelamotic melanomas) and because tissues other than melanin, such as blood breakdown products, can also cause relaxation enhancement.

Treatment is based on the size, location, and extent of the tumor. Brachytherapy with or without local excision, enucleation, orbital exenteration, or percutaneous proton irradiation are all treatment options.

SUGGESTED READINGS

Gomori JM, et al. Choroidal melanomas: correlation of NMR spectroscopy and MR imaging. *Radiology* 1986;158:443–445.

Mafee MF. Malignant uveal melanoma and simulating lesions. MR imaging evaluation. *Radiology* 1986;160:773–780.

Potter PD, Shields CL, Shields JA, et al. The role of magnetic resonance imaging in children with intraocular tumors and simulating lesions. *Ophthalmology* 1996;103:1774–1783.

Romani A, Baldeschi L, Genovesi-Ebert F, et al. Sensitivity and specificity of ultrasonography, fluorescein videoangiography, indocyanine green videoangiography, magnetic resonance and radioimmunoscintigraphy in the diagnosis of primary choroidal malignant melanoma. *Ophthalmologica* 1998;212(Suppl 1):44–46.

Scott IU, Murray TG, Hughes JR. Evaluation of imaging techniques for detection of extraocular extension of choroidal melanoma. *Arch Ophthalmol* 1998;116:897–899.

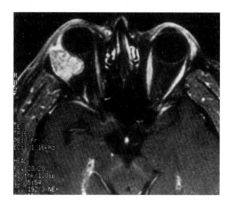

FIGURE 42.1A

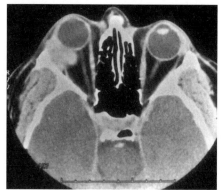

FIGURE 42.1B

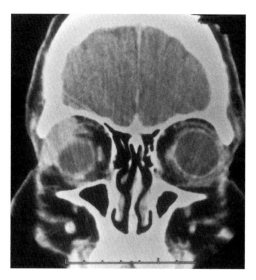

FIGURE 42.1C

CLINICAL HISTORY

The patient is an adult male with new onset proptosis on the right.

FINDINGS

The axial MR images show mild right proptosis with enlargement of the right lacrimal gland. The gland signal intensity is high signal (Fig. 42.1A). There is no evidence of invasion of surrounding structures. The CT axial and coronal views confirm that the mass is arising from the lacrimal gland (Fig. 42.1B, C).

DIAGNOSIS

Lacrimal gland enlargement resulting from adenocarcinoma.

DISCUSSION

Enlargement of the lacrimal gland is usually a nonspecific radiographic finding that may be due to either inflammatory (dacroadenitis) or neoplastic conditions. The lacrimal glands may be involved with a variety of disease processes. However, because of the histologic similarities of the lacrimal gland with salivary gland tissue, these two groups of glands share many of the same pathologies. Although the radiologic findings are usually nonspecific, the clinical setting may help suggest the diagnosis.

One useful approach to diagnosing masses of the lacrimal glands is to consider that approximately 50% are of the lymphoid/inflammatory type and 50% are epithelial cell tumors. Dermoid cysts are not included in this scheme because, although dermoid cysts may arise near the lacrimal fossa, they are not true lacrimal gland lesions but instead arise from embryologic rests in the orbit. Metastases to the lacrimal gland have been reported but are rare.

Radiographically, epithelial cell tumors are more likely to show aggressive behavior and occasionally bone involvement. Half of the tumors in this group are pleomorphic adenomas. The remaining 50% include adenoid cystic carcinoma, mucoepidermoid carcinoma, adenocarcinoma, and others.

The other half of masses in the lacrimal gland are in the lymphoid/inflammatory group. They run the spectrum from mild inflammatory conditions to lymphoma (usually non-Hodgkin's). Lesions in this group tend to result in diffuse enlargement of the gland and usually show no bone erosion.

It is useful to group these lesions according to their time course. The acute group includes bacterial and viral dacroadenitis and tends to involve younger age groups. Orbital pseudotumor and lymphoma can also present with this picture. Entities in the acute group can also have a more chronic course.

Other more chronic conditions to be considered are sarcoid, Wegener's, thyroid ophthalmopathy, Mikulicz's, and Sjögren's syndrome. Mikulicz's syndrome is nonspecific lacrimal (and salivary) gland swelling associated with leukemia, lymphoma, tuberculosis, syphilis, and sarcoid.

Clinical management of lacrimal gland masses depends on the pathology involved. Although a specific tissue diagnosis is often not possible based of the CT or MR findings, these studies provide valuable information about the extent of disease and involvement of adjacent structures.

SUGGESTED READINGS

Bilaniuk LT, Farber M. Imaging of developmental anomalies of the eye and the orbit. *AJNR Am J Neuroradiol* 1992;13:793–803.

Carmody RF, Mafee MF, Goodwin JA, et al. Orbital and optic pathway sarcoidosis: MR findings. *AJNR Am J Neuroradiol* 1994;15:775–783.

Krzystolik M, Warner MA. Orbit and adnexal neoplasia. *Curr Opin Ophthalmol* 1995;6:78–85.

Shields CL, Shields JA. Lacrimal gland tumors. *Int Ophthalmol Clin* 1993;33:181–188.

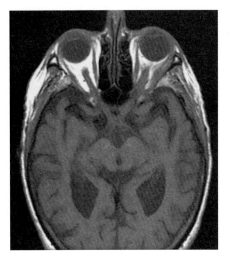

FIGURE 43.1A

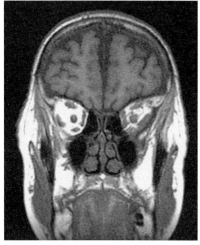

FIGURE 43.1B

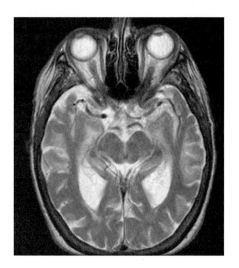

FIGURE 43.1C

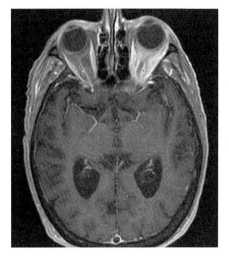

FIGURE 43.1D

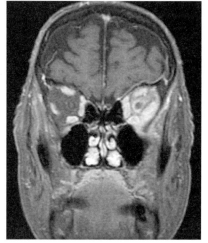

FIGURE 43.1E

CLINICAL HISTORY

An elderly woman presents with acute orbital pain. On clinical examination, there is no proptosis and no inflammatory changes noted in the anterior orbital compartment.

FINDINGS

Axial and coronal T1-weighted MR images of the orbits show enlargement of the extraocular muscles (EOMs) on the left, including the tendinous attachments to the globe (Fig. 43.1A, B). The margins of the muscles are ill defined. T2-weighted images show a similar pattern (Fig. 43.1C).

Axial and coronal T1-weighted images postcontrast show abnormal enhancement of the extraocular muscles, intraconal fat, and along the optic nerve sheath. These changes are more pronounced in the orbital apex (Fig. 43.1D, E).

DIAGNOSIS

Orbital pseudotumor.

DISCUSSION

The term orbital pseudotumor describes an idiopathic inflammatory condition involving the orbit. It is the third most common ophthalmologic disease after thyroid orbitopathy and lymphoproliferative disorders, and it is the most frequent cause of an intraorbital mass in adults. It is the underlying cause of unilateral exophthalmos in 25% of patients. Only 5% to 15% of cases of orbital pseudotumor present in the pediatric age group.

The symptoms in orbital pseudotumor depend on the degree of inflammatory response, the stage (acute, subacute, or chronic), and on the affected orbital structures. The most common symptoms in the acute inflammatory form of disease include abrupt onset of orbital pain, swelling of the periorbital tissues, double vision, and, occasionally, decreased vision. This form of presentation is easily confused with orbital or periorbital infection, and it is not unusual that patients are initially given antibiotics for several days. Patients typically present with ophthalmoplegia, diplopia, proptosis, and progressive visual loss.

Orbital pseudotumor is often classified into six categories: (a) acute and subacute idiopathic anterior orbital pseudotumor, (b) acute and subacute idiopathic diffuse orbital inflammation, (c) myositic form, (d) apical orbital inflammation (Tolosa-Hunt syndrome), (e) idiopathic dacryoadenitis, and (f) idiopathic perineuritis. The Tolosa-Hunt syndrome is a variant of pseudotumor characterized by an inflammatory infiltration of the orbital apex, with extension into the superior orbital fissure and cavernous sinus. Clinically it manifests by painful ophthalmoplegia involving cranial nerves III, IV, and VI and hypesthesia of the periorbital tissues as a result of involvement of the first division of the trigeminal nerve.

Orbital pseudotumor defines a clinically and histologically heterogeneous group of lesions for which an identifiable cause cannot be found. It is a diagnosis of exclusion, after other local or systemic disease processes with similar clinicoradiographic findings have been ruled out. Proposed etiologic factors include an autoimmune process and lymphoproliferative disease. Histologic changes define two different types of orbital pseudotumor and may vary in the course of the disease. In the acute inflammatory type, there is infiltration of the orbit by polymorphous acute inflammatory cells dispersed in a matrix of granulation tissue, whereas in the chronic sclerosing form, inflammatory changes are replaced by fibrotic tissue with subsequent stretching and deformity of the intraorbital structures. There is also a predominantly lymphocytic variety of pseudotumor, thought to be a prelymphomatous condition.

Imaging of orbital pseudotumor, although nonspecific, is useful in defining the extent of the disease and excluding true orbital tumors. When the differentiation from orbital tumor is not possible, fine-needle aspiration (FNA) may be required. CT and MRI are best suited for these goals, with MRI being superior to CT in the evaluation of the optic nerve, cavernous sinus, and globe. Fat-saturated T1-weighted sequences after contrast enhancement are required for evaluation of inflammatory changes in the retrobulbar fat, optic nerve, and cavernous sinus. Ocular ultrasound is a good method to evaluate the globe but is much less accurate for assessment of the retrobulbar structures. The structures involved by orbital pseudotumor are, in decreasing order of frequency, retrobulbar fat (76%), extraocular muscles (57%), optic nerve (38%), uvea and sclera (33%), and lacrimal gland (5%).

In general terms, the most important imaging features in differentiating pseudotumor from true neoplastic disease are the absence of mass effect, confinement to the space of origin, and the lack of bony destruction. However, there are a few reported cases of extraorbital extension of pseudotumor, including intracranial extension. As opposed to lymphoma, orbital pseudotumor shows intense enhancement and is hyperintense on T2-weighted images (except for the sclerosing variety). When the diagnosis is in doubt, imaging guided FNA, followed by flow cytometry or Southern blot analysis of the cytopathologic specimen, usually allows differentiation between the lymphocytic variety of pseudotumor and true lymphoma.

Orbital pseudotumor usually has a dramatic and rapid response to steroids. However, other diseases, including tumors, may have a partial response to steroids. The acute inflammatory variety of the disease is particularly sensitive to steroids. The subacute and chronic forms, including the sclerosing variety, are unresponsive. Radiation therapy and immunosuppressors may be used in patients unresponsive to steroids, but are not successful in treating fibrosclerosing lesions. When the optic nerve is in danger of compressive ischemic neuropathy, surgical decompression should be attempted.

SUGGESTED READINGS

Atabay C, Tyutyunikov A, Scalise D, et al. Serum antibodies reactive with eye muscle membrane antigens are detected in patients with nonspecific orbital inflammation. *Ophthalmology* 1995;102:145–153.

Berger JW, Rubin PA, Jakobiec FA. Pediatric orbital pseudotumor: case report and review of the literature. Int Ophthalmol Clin 1996;36:161–177.

Char DH, Miller T. Orbital pseudotumor. Fine-needle aspiration biopsy and response to therapy. *Ophthalmology* 1993;100:1702–1710.

de Jesus O, Inserni JA, Gonzalez A, et al. Idiopathic orbital inflammation with intracranial extension. Case report. *J Neurosurg* 1996;85:510–513.

Mombaerts I, Goldschmeding R, Schlingemann RO, et al. What is orbital pseudotumor? Surv Ophthalmol 1996;41:66–78.

Mombaerts I, Schlingemann RO, Goldschmeding R, et al. Are systemic corticosteroids useful in the management of orbital pseudotumors? *Ophthalmology* 1996;103:521–528.

Mombaerts I, Schlingemann RO, Goldschmeding R, et al. Idiopathic granulomatous orbital inflammation. *Ophthalmology* 1996;103:2135–2141.

Notter M, Kern T, Forrer A, et al. Radiotherapy of pseudotumor orbitae. *Front Radiat Ther Oncol* 1997;30:180–191.

Osguthorpe JD, Hochman M. Inflammatory sinus diseases affecting the orbit. *Otolaryngol Clin North Am* 1993;26:657–671.

Weber AL, Jakobiec FA, Sabates NR. Pseudotumor of the orbit. *Neuroimag Clin North Am* 1996;6:73–92.

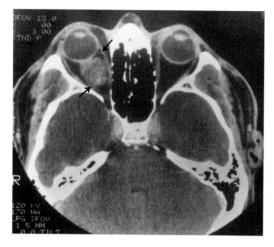

FIGURE 44.1A

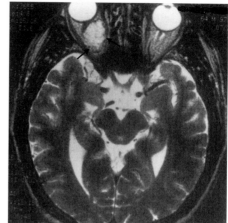

FIGURE 44.1B

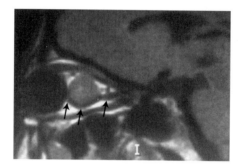

FIGURE 44.1C

CLINICAL HISTORY

A 60-year-old man presents with gradual proptosis of the right globe over several years.

FINDINGS

A well-defined mass in the intraconal space is present on the axial CT scan on the right (Fig. 44.1A). The axial T2-weighted MR image shows homogeneous increased signal intensity throughout the mass (Fig. 44.1B). The mass effect causes a slight proptosis. The sagittal T1-weighted image shows that the mass displaces the optic nerve inferiorly (Fig. 44.1C). (Image courtesy Drs. Andrew Berger and Ed Helmer).

DIAGNOSIS

Cavernous hemangioma.

DISCUSSION

Cavernous hemangioma is one of the most common tumors of the orbit and the most common benign primary orbital tumor in the adult. There is a female preponderance, and it usually presents in the third to fifth decades of life. The majority of cavernous hemangiomas are solitary.

The clinical course is characteristic: a slow, progressive enlargement with findings related to displacement or compression of orbital structures. This is in distinction to capillary hemangiomas, which tend to decrease in size over time. The sign or symptom at the time of diagnosis is usually proptosis. If the tumor is in the orbital apex, it may produce diplopia and optic nerve compression.

Cavernous hemangiomas are round or oval in shape and may have a slightly nodular surface. Macroscopically, they are purplish red in color, well circumscribed, and encapsulated by a fine fibrous capsule. Microscopically, cavernous hemangiomas have numerous blood-filled vascular channels that are lined with flattened endothelial cells that are surrounded by smooth muscle. The vascular channels are often separated by fibrous septa. Rarely, phleboliths may be present. Intramuscular hemangiomas may also occasionally occur.

Typical MR and CT appearance is that of an oval or round, well-defined enhancing tumor in the intraconal space. The mass is soft and conforms to the shape of the orbit without distorting that structure. Occasionally, a small portion of the lesion may extend into the extraconal space.

On MRI, it is usually homogeneous in intensity on T1-weighted sequences and heterogeneous in appearance on T2-weighted images. On a T1-weighted image, the intensity is greater than muscle and globe and much less than fat. On a T2-weighted image, it is more intense than any other tissue. The marked hyperintensity on T2 weighting is due to the high fluid content of the numerous blood-filled microscopic spaces. This fluid component predominates over that of the fibrous and supporting tissues and results in marked hyperintensity. Enhancement with contrast agents occurs diffusely and moderately. A cavernous hemangioma grows insidiously and may become so large that it can expand and remodel the orbital walls.

Surgical excision is the treatment of choice. The encapsulated tumor can easily be totally removed. Cavernous hemangiomas generally do not recur even after incomplete excision.

SUGGESTED READINGS

Bilaniuk LT, Rapoport RJ. Magnetic resonance imaging of the orbit. *Top Magn Reson Imaging* 1994;6:167–181.

Forbes G. Vascular lesions in the orbit. *Neuroimag Clin North Am* 1996;6:113–222.

Mukherji SK, Tart RP, Fitzsimmons J, et al. Fat-suppressed MR of the orbit and cavernous sinus: comparison of fast spin-echo and conventional spin-echo. *AJNR Am J Neuroradiol* 1994;15:1707—1714.

Sweet C, Silbergleit R, Mehta B. Primary intraosseous hemangioma of the orbit: CT and MR appearance. *AJNR Am J Neuroradiol* 1997;18:379—381.

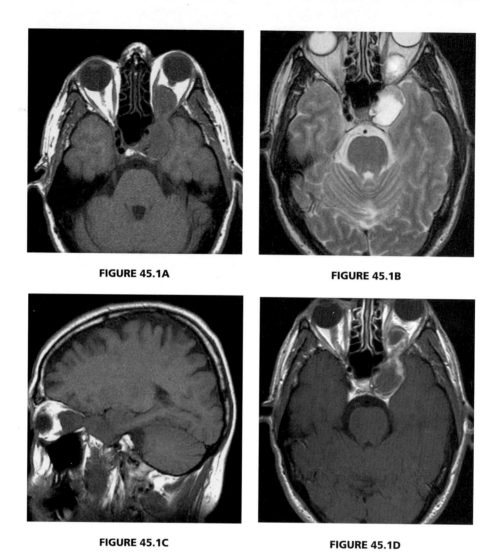

FIGURE 45.1A

FIGURE 45.1B

FIGURE 45.1C

FIGURE 45.1D

CLINICAL HISTORY

A 50-year-old woman presents with progressive loss of vision in her left eye. Physical examination reveals proptosis and impaired mobility of the left globe.

FINDINGS

There is a large hourglass-shaped mass with a larger component centered in the left cavernous sinus and a smaller intraorbital component on the axial T1-weighted images (Fig. 45.1A). It is heterogeneous on T2-weighted image (Fig. 45.1B). The mass extends into the orbit through the optic canal, which is markedly enlarged (Fig. 45.1C). The cavernous segment of the ICA is medially displaced and compressed by this lesion. The postcontrast images show peripheral enhancement (Fig. 45.1D).

DIAGNOSIS

Intraorbital meningioma with extension to the cavernous sinus.

DISCUSSION

Optic nerve meningiomas comprise 5% to 7% of all primary orbital tumors. Females are more frequently affected than males (4:1) and, although there is a broad range, a peak incidence is seen in the fourth and fifth decades. Intraorbital meningiomas can also occur in children, usually in the first decade of life, and show more aggressive behavior than the adult form. Bilateral meningiomas are a diagnostic criteria for neurofibromatosis type 1.

Intraorbital meningiomas may originate within the orbit or rarely result from direct extension of an intracranial tumor usually arising from the sphenoid ridge. Intraorbital meningiomas can arise from the meningeal sheath of the optic nerve or from remnants of meningoepithelial cells left behind during embryologic development. The most common location is the optic nerve sheath and the orbital apex. However, meningiomas of the extraconal compartment can be seen, usually arising from the periosteum of the orbital walls. Intracranial meningiomas gain access to the orbit either by extension along neural and vascular foramina or through invasion of the bony walls of the orbit.

The clinical presentation of intraorbital meningiomas is nonspecific, similar to any other intraorbital mass. The most frequent presenting symptoms include decreased vision, proptosis, and constriction of the visual field. However, the clinical presentation largely depends on the size and location of the tumor. Small meningiomas arising along the optic nerve sheath may be asymptomatic for long periods before they come to clinical attention.

CT and MRI have complementary roles in the evaluation of intraorbital masses. Although MRI has superior soft tissue contrast resolution, in the case of an intraorbital meningioma, CT is superior in detecting intratumoral calcification and associated bony changes which may be important clues in the differential diagnosis. Beam hardening artifact caused by adjacent bone is one limitation of CT, particularly in the evaluation of small perioptic meningiomas.

MRI is more accurate in the detection of optic nerve–sheath complex enlargement, especially when enhanced coronal T1-weighted images with fat saturation are performed. This sequence provides better contrast resolution between the enhancing lesion and the intraconal fat (also hyperintense on T1-weighted image) and is crucial in the diagnosis of small perioptic tumors. Orbital meningiomas are usually slightly hypointense to the brain parenchyma on both T1- and T2-weighted images, and enhance vividly and homogeneously, being clearly distinguishable from the optic nerve. Coronal images are particularly well suited for evaluation of the optic canal, the optic chiasm, and the precise relationship between the lesion and the optic nerve.

Meningiomas are well circumscribed unless they breach the dural lining and infiltrate the surrounding fat. This is seen more frequently in pediatric patients and represents more aggressive behavior. Associated bony sclerosis may be depicted on MRI as an enlarged area of absent signal corresponding to the enlarged cortical bone.

Diffuse enhancement along the optic nerve is more likely to be related to an inflammatory process, although sometimes impossible to distinguish from tumor.

The management of lesions involving the anterior optic pathways is controversial. The treatment of intraorbital meningiomas depends upon their location, extent, and associated symptoms. As opposed to nerve sheath meningiomas, extradural or "ectopic" meningiomas are usually easy to resect without endangering the optic pathway. Intracanalicular and nerve sheath meningiomas, with some rare exceptions, are not amenable to complete resection without considerable risk of optic nerve damage as a result of the close proximity of the ophthalmic and central retinal arteries. Surgery is indicated when there is loss of visual acuity, increased proptosis, pain, or radiographic evidence of further growth. Intracranial lesions with intraorbital extension require a multidisciplinary approach with surgery performed by a team of neurosurgeons and skull base surgeons.

SUGGESTED READINGS

Biesman BS, Heilman C. Surgical management of lesions affecting the anterior optic pathways. *Semin Ophthalmol* 1995;10:260–264.

Delfini R, Missori P, Tarantino R, et al. Primary benign tumors of the orbital cavity: comparative data in a series of patients with optic nerve glioma, sheath meningioma, or neurinoma. *Surg Neurol* 1996;45:147–153; discussion 153–154.

Gunalp I, Gunduz K, Duruk K, et al. Neurogenic tumors of the orbit. *Jpn J Ophthalmol* 1994;38:185–190.

Hashimoto M, Tomura N, Watarai J. Retrobulbar orbital metastasis mimicking meningioma. *Radiat Med* 1995;13:77–79.

Ing EB, Garrity JA, Cross SA, et al. Sarcoid masquerading as optic nerve sheath meningioma. *Mayo Clin Proc* 1997;72:38–43.

Johnson TE, Weatherhead RG, Nasr AM, et al. Ectopic (extradural) meningioma of the orbit: a report of two cases in children. *J Pediatr Ophthalmol Strabismus* 1993;30:43–47.

Miller NR, Golnik KC, Zeidman SM, et al. Pneumosinus dilatans: a sign of intracranial meningioma. *Surg Neurol* 1996;46:471–474.

Reid D, Ngo HH, Lamarche JB. Primary post-traumatic intraorbital meningioma. *J Otolaryngol* 1994;23:298–301.

Rose GE. Orbital meningiomas: surgery, radiotherapy, or hormones? *Br J Ophthalmol* 1993;77:313–314.

Ruscalleda J, Feliciani M, Avila A, et al. Neuroradiological features of intracranial and intraorbital meningeal hemangiopericytomas. *Neurodiology* 1994;36:440–445.

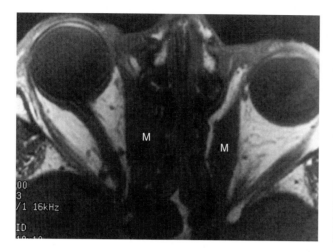

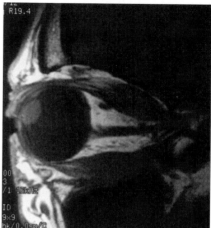

FIGURE 46.1A　　　　　　　　**FIGURE 46.1B**

CLINICAL HISTORY

A 48-year-old woman presents with progressive bilateral painless exophthalmus.

FINDINGS

Axial surface coil MRI of the orbits shows enlargement of the muscular bellies of the medial recti, sparing the tendinous insertions in the globe. There is some crowding of the orbital apices but a thin rim of fat is seen surrounding both optic nerves. There has been prior orbital decompression with partial resection of the lamina papyracea bilaterally (Fig. 46.1A). A mild degree of proptosis is noted. The coronal view shows similar enlargement of the superior and inferior recti as well (Fig. 46.1B).

DIAGNOSIS

Thyroid orbitopathy.

DISCUSSION

Thyroid orbitopathy is also referred to as thyroid-associated ophthalmopathy, autoimmune thyroid disease, endocrine exophthalmus, and Graves' ophthalmopathy. It is the most common orbital disorder, affecting approximately 0.5% of the US population. Thyroid orbitopathy is the most frequent cause of exophthalmus in adults, representing 80% of bilateral and 15% to 28% of unilateral exophthalmus. It usually presents in adulthood with a peak incidence in the fourth and fifth decades of life. Only 5% of cases occur before age 15 years. Females are more frequently affected.

The extraocular muscles (EOM) are the most common orbital structures to be affected. The involvement is bilateral in 70% to 85% of cases, although asymmetric in 20% to 30%. Isolated involvement of a single EOM is much less common, only seen in 10% of patients.

Hyperthyroidism is present in the majority of patients (70%), with increased levels of T3 and T4. However, thyroid ophthalmopathy may be the first sign of Graves' disease and precede any hormonal changes by a year or more. The incidence of proptosis varies widely in different series, ranging from 35% to 93%.

Thyroid ophthalmopathy is due to deposition of abnormal material in the orbital contents, predominantly involving the EOM and retrobulbar fat. This process is thought to have an autoimmune origin as a result of cross-reactivity between the eye muscle and thyroid autoantigens. Several autoantibodies have been implicated, including LATS (long-acting thyroid-stimulating factor) and TSI (thyroid-stimulating immunoglobulins), which are now recognized as antibodies against the thyrotropin receptors of the thyroid gland.

The degree of orbital involvement does not correlate with the degree of thyroid dysfunction or the levels of circulating LATS. The most common presenting symptoms are proptosis and double vision. Blindness from ischemic optic neuropathy is a dismal consequence of thyroid orbitopathy if early decompression is not undertaken. Corneal ulceration, due to exposure keratitis, is another possible complication of the disease. A family history should be elicited, because 30% of patients have other familial autoimmune disorders.

Ultrasonography, CT, and MRI may be used to evaluate orbital involvement in Graves' disease. Because orbital involvement may be subclinical, all patients should have an imaging study as a screening test for thyroid orbitopathy. Imaging is useful for detection and serial follow up of proptosis and is crucial for detection of optic nerve compression. The degree of proptosis is measured in the axial plane at the level of the lens, from the interzygomatic line to the anterior margin of the globe.

The major finding on cross-sectional imaging is enlargement and enhancement of the EOM, which is usually bilateral and asymmetric. Typically, the muscles most frequently involved are, in decreasing order of frequency, the inferior, medial, superior, and lateral rectus. In patients with isolated involvement of a single muscle, the superior rectus and levator palpebrae complex is most commonly affected. Classi-cally, the swelling is maximal in the belly of the muscle, sparing the tendinous attachment to the globe, and the margins of the involved muscles are smooth. These are important distinguishing features from orbital pseudotumor, which usually involves the entire length of the muscle and shows ill-defined margins. Other CT findings include increased volume and increased density of the retrobulbar fat and uveoscleral thickening.

On MRI, the enlarged muscles are hyperintense on T2-weighted images as a result of edema and inflammation. Fat-saturated enhanced T1-weighted images are very sensitive for detection of muscle enlargement caused by the increased vascularity of the muscle. The better contrast resolution of MRI makes it the best method to evaluate for optic nerve compression. A "tram track" sign on T2-weighted images may be seen representing dilatation of the subarachnoid space surrounding the optic nerve and is suspicious for optic nerve compression. Differential diagnosis of this sign includes increased intracranial pressure and pseudotumor cerebri.

Left to its natural course, the disease resolves spontaneously in the majority of patients. However, in 10% of cases the progression of orbital involvement leads to recurrent corneal ulcerations and loss of vision. Immunosuppressive drugs have been used with varying success rates, although the inherent risks of this kind of therapy limits their use in this benign condition. Surgery is the only successful therapy in the chronic fibrotic stage of the disease and may be used to correct eyelid retraction or to decompress the optic nerve. Surgical procedures attempt to increase the bony orbit or remove orbital fat in order to decompress the orbital contents.

SUGGESTED READINGS

Cangiarella J, Cajigas A, Savala E, et al. Fine needle aspiration cytology of orbital masses. *Acta Cytologica* 1996;40:1205–1211.

Kao SC, Kendler DL, Nugent RA, et al. Radiotherapy in the management of thyroid orbitopathy. Computed tomography and clinical outcomes. *Arch Ophthalmol* 1993;111:819–823.

McNab AA. Orbital decompression for thyroid orbitopathy. *Aust N Z J Ophthalmol* 1997;25:55–61.

Postema PT, Krenning EP, Wijngaarde R, et al. ^{111}In-DTPA-D-Phe1 octreotide scintigraphy in thyroidal and orbital Graves' disease: a parameter for disease activity? *J Clin Endocrinol Metab* 1994;79:1845–1851.

Rosen CE, Kennerdell JS. Extreme eyelid swelling as an unusual presentation of dysthyroid orbitopathy. *J Neurooph-thalmol* 1995;15:84–89.

Sendrowski DP. Hyperthyroidism. *Optom Clin* 1994;3:87–97.

Shokeir MO, Pudek MR, Katz S, et al. The relationship of thyrotropin receptor antibody levels to the severity of thyroid orbitopathy. *Clin Biochem* 1996;29:187–189.

Villadolid MC, Yokoyama N, Izumi M, et al. Untreated Graves' disease in patients without clinical ophthalmopathy demonstrate a high frequency of extraocular muscle enlargement. *J Clin Endocrinol Metab* 1995;80:2830–2833.

Weber A, Dallow R, Sabates N. Graves' disease of the orbit. *Neuroimag Clin North Am* 1996;6:61–72.

Wilson WB, Prochoda M. Radiotherapy for thyroid orbitopathy. Effects on extraocular muscle balance. *Arch Ophthalmol* 1995;13:1420–1425.

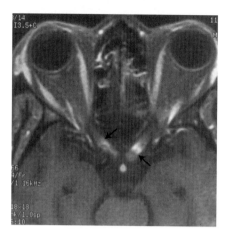

FIGURE 47.1A

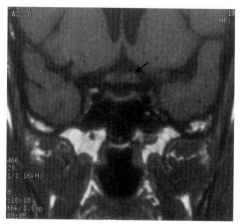

FIGURE 47.1B

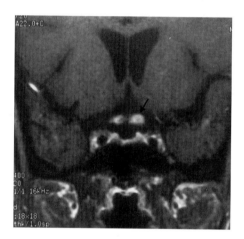

FIGURE 47.1C

CLINICAL HISTORY

The patient is a 48-year-old woman with a history of prior surgery and radiation therapy for a left frontal lobe neoplasm who presented with new onset of decreased visual acuity.

FINDINGS

Axial postcontrast frequency selective fat suppression imaging (FATSAT) T1-weighted image shows enlargement and abnormal enhancement of the retrocanalicular segment of the optic nerves, left greater than right (Fig. 47.1A). Coronal noncontrast T1-weighted image of the orbits shows enlargement of the retrocanalicular segments of the optic nerves as they join the chiasm (Fig. 47.1B). Coronal postcontrast FATSAT T1-weighted image shows enlargement and abnormal enhancement of the retrocanalicular segments of the optic nerves and optic chiasm, left greater than right (Fig. 47.1C).

DIAGNOSIS

Radiation-induced optic neuropathy.

DISCUSSION

Optic neuritis is a general term used to describe an acute inflammatory condition involving the optic nerve, usually presenting as rapid onset of visual loss. Although it occurs as an isolated entity, its greater significance results from its association with multiple sclerosis (MS). In fact, the term *optic neuritis* is often misused as a synonym of optic nerve involvement in MS. Optic neuritis is a relatively common disease affecting young adults (mean age of 30 years). There is a slight female predominance. The disease is rare in children.

Optic neuritis may be asymptomatic, although typically patients present with sudden loss of visual acuity, pain with eye movement, and dyschromatopsia. Symptoms are unilateral in 70% of cases. Diagnosis is based on clinical history and ophthalmologic evaluation including assessment of visual acuity, color vision, and visual fields.

A thorough clinical history and neurologic examination should be performed in order to exclude MS. Even when optic neuritis is seen in isolation, patients should be closely followed up because MS will eventually develop in a significant percentage.

Optic nerve inflammation may be due to multiple pathologic processes including demyelinating disease, infection, systemic inflammatory processes, optic nerve ischemia, and toxic insults. Because the optic nerve is an extension of the central nervous system (CNS), consisting of bundles of myelinated axons, it is not surprising that it is involved by the same demyelinating diseases as the brain. MS develops in approximately 35% to 40% of patients with MS and, in 15% to 20%, optic neuritis is the initial manifestation of MS, meaning that MS develops in 20% of patients with optic neuritis over a short or longer term. Concurrent optic neuritis and cervical myelitis is known as Devicz's syndrome and is uncommonly seen in patients with MS.

Infectious processes involving the central nervous system and meninges may spread to the optic nerve. The conduit for spread may be the nerve itself (neurotropic viruses such as human immunodeficiency virus) or the cerebrospinal fluid in the optic nerve sheath. Basilar meningitides such as tuberculosis and fungal meningitis are the most common infectious processes spreading to the optic nerve.

Systemic vasculopathies of small and medium sized vessels may also be responsible for optic neuritis.

The optic nerve is fairly sensitive to radiation injury and radiation necrosis of the optic nerve is a well-known complication when the optic nerve is included in the radiation field. This is usually encountered after radiotherapy for orbital, sinonasal, sellar, and orbitofrontal neoplasms. The effects of radiation are dependent both in the total dose and the amount of fractionation.

Abnormal imaging findings are not required for the diagnosis of optic neuritis and, when present, the findings are nonspecific. The main role of imaging is to exclude other pathologic processes and to detect other white matter abnormalities in the CNS, making the diagnosis of MS more likely. Imaging is also important in the evaluation of treatment efficacy and in long-term follow-up.

The best imaging modality to evaluate the visual pathway is MRI. The study should include the orbits and brain. Postcontrast fat-suppressed axial and coronal T1-weighted images of the orbits are mandatory. The most common findings are optic nerve enlargement and optic nerve enhancement, which may be focal, segmental, or diffuse. Single or multiple discontinuous lesions may be seen. More nodular enhancement suggests neoplastic involvement, although sarcoid and some infectious processes (such as tuberculosis and fungal infection) may have a similar appearance. MRI may also show T2-weighted hyperintensity in the optic nerve, optic chiasm, and in the parenchymal white matter.

T2-weighted abnormality or optic nerve enhancement is present in 56% to 72% of patients with isolated optic neuritis and in 90% to 98% of patients with definitive MS.

Radiation necrosis manifests as a focally expanded, enhancing optic nerve and optic chiasm. Contrast enhancement is thought to be due to vascular injury resulting in increased permeability of the blood–brain barrier.

Steroids are used as the "gold standard" treatment for optic neuritis, regardless of cause. Several studies have shown a more rapid recovery of vision and a transient protective effect from development of MS with the use of intravenous methylprednisolone.

SUGGESTED READINGS

Cornblath WT, Quint DJ. MRI of optic nerve enlargement in optic neuritis. *Neurology* 1997;48:821–825.

Kortvelesy S. Recent advances in the management of optic neuritis. *Hawaii Med J* 1997;56:281.

Villablanca P, Curran J, Arnold A, et al. Orbit and optic nerve. *Top Magn Res Imag* 1996;8:87–110.

Weber AL, Klufas R, Pless M. Imaging evaluation of the optic nerve and visual pathway including cranial nerves affecting the visual pathway. *Neuroimag Clin North Am* 1996;6:143–177.

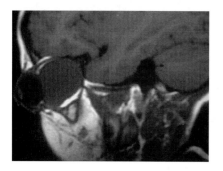 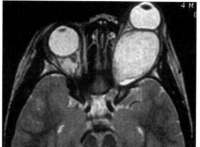 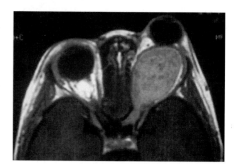

FIGURE 48.1A　　　　　**FIGURE 48.1B**　　　　　**FIGURE 48.1C**

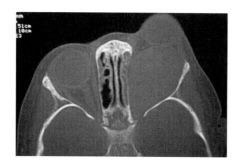 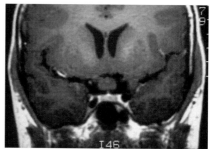

FIGURE 48.2　　　　　**FIGURE 48.3**

CLINICAL HISTORY

A 4-year-old boy presents with left-sided proptosis and decreased vision.

FINDINGS

Sagittal T1-weighted, axial T2-weighted, and axial postgadolinium T1-weighted images through the orbits (Figs. 48.1A–C) show a large, smooth, fusiform mass involving the left optic nerve and extending through the optic canal into the prechiasmatic segment of the nerve abutting the chiasm (best seen on the contrast-enhanced axial T1-weighted image). The mass is isointense to gray matter on the T1-weighted image and hyperintense on the T2-weighted image, and it enhances homogeneously without areas of cystic degeneration or hemorrhage. There is marked proptosis and inward deformity of the posterior aspect of the left globe by this mass, which is seen on the sagittal T1-weighted image. The right optic nerve is normal in appearance.

Axial CT section through the optic canal (bone window) shows enlargement and remodeling of the bony orbit with inward bowing of the lamina papyracea and enlargement of the optic canal when compared with the contralateral side (Fig. 48.2).

Coronal postgadolinium T1-weighted images show enlargement of the chiasm and prechiasmatic segments of both optic nerves (Fig. 48.3, another patient). There is no associated enhancement.

DIAGNOSIS

Optic nerve glioma.

DISCUSSION

Optic nerve gliomas account for 3% of all intraorbital tumors and are thought to arise from the neuroglia of the optic nerve. In children, they are almost always low-grade, slow-growing tumors classified as grade I astrocytomas. The adult forms are more variable in histology and usually represent intraorbital extension of intracranial gliomas originating in the chiasm or retrochiasmatic optic pathway. These tumors can involve several segments of the retrobulbar visual pathway including the optic nerve, chiasm, optic tracts, geniculate bodies, and optic radiations. Tumors confined to the intraorbital optic nerve are rare.

Ninety percent of optic gliomas are diagnosed in children younger than 10 years and the peak incidence is between ages 2 and 6 years. Fifteen percent of patients with optic gliomas have neurofibromatosis type I, and, not uncommonly, gliomas are the first sign of the disease. Bilateral optic nerve gliomas are pathognomonic of neurofibromatosis type I and occur in 5% to 15% of cases.

Painless proptosis is the most frequent form of presentation. Patients may also have peripheral constriction of the visual field and episodes of transient visual obscuration that progress to decreased vision and, eventually, to blindness. Optic atrophy and disc edema are the most common funduscopic findings. A few clinical features may help in differentiating optic nerve gliomas from optic sheath meningiomas. Loss of vision in the first decade, mild proptosis with significant visual impairment, and transient obscuration of vision in extreme gaze or with changes in head position all favor the diagnosis of optic glioma. However, the most important factor in the differential diagnosis is age: optic sheath meningiomas are more frequent than optic gliomas in adult patients whereas they are rare tumors in the pediatric age group. In optic gliomas, blindness is the combined result of vascular ischemia and disorganization of the nerve structure by proliferative astrocytes.

Imaging is very useful in the differential diagnosis of intraorbital lesions and in determining the extent of neoplastic processes. Optic nerve gliomas are smoothly marginated, fusiform-shaped tumors, usually along the axis of the nerve and are confined by its dural covering. When large enough, they lead to proptosis and may typically indent the posterior surface of the globe. On MRI, the tumor is isointense to gray matter on T1-weighted images and hyperintense on T2-weighted images. Enhancement is variable and depends on tumor location. Whereas purely intraorbital tumors tend to have minimal or no enhancement, tumors arising in the optic chiasm and retrochiasmatic visual pathway tend to enhance moderately to intensely. Cystic changes may be seen as a result of intracellular and extracellular mucinous components whereas calcification is not a feature of these tumors. Large tumors may remodel the bony orbit and enlarge the optic canal, best seen on CT (see Fig. 2). MR is the best modality to determine the extent of tumor beyond the orbit to the prechiasmatic optic nerve, chiasm, and retrochiasmatic visual pathway.

Optic gliomas may be difficult to manage. Because both forms of therapy, surgery and radiation, may lead to blindness, treatment is usually postponed until there is visual loss. However, in unilateral tumors growing toward the chiasm, treatment is mandatory to save vision in the contralateral eye.

SUGGESTED READINGS

Biesman BS, Heilman C. Surgical management of lesions affecting the anterior optic pathways. *Semin Ophthalmol* 1995;10:260–264.

Delfini R, Missori P, Tarantino R, et al. Primary benign tumors of the orbital cavity: comparative data in a series of patients with optic nerve glioma, sheath meningioma and neurinoma. *Surg Neurol* 1996;45:147–153.

Hoyt WF, Bagdhassarian SA. Optic glioma of childhood. Natural history and rationale for conservative management. *Br J Ophthalmol* 1989;53:793–798.

Mohadjer M. Chiasmatic optic glioma. *Neurochirurgia (Stuttgart)* 1991;34:90–93.

Wright JE. Optic nerve glioma and the management of optic nerve tumours in the young. *Br J Ophthalmol* 1989;73:967–974.

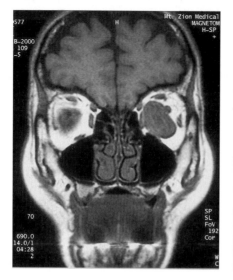

FIGURE 49.1

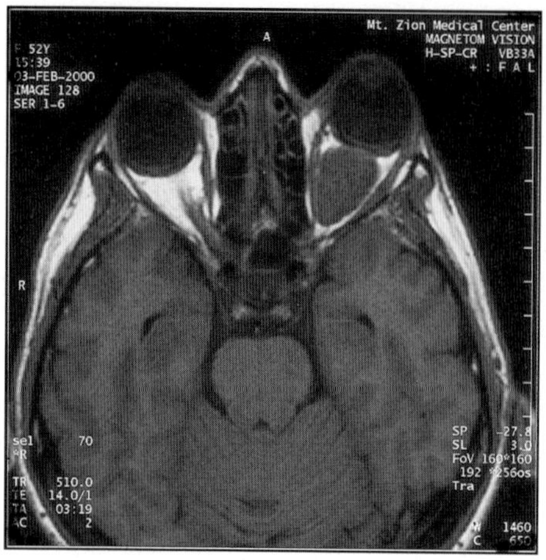

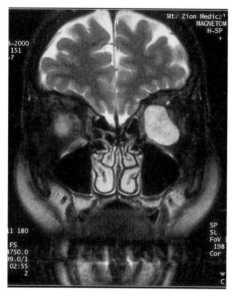

FIGURE 49.3

FIGURE 49.2

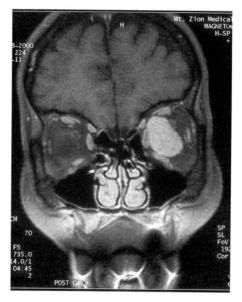

FIGURE 49.4

CLINICAL HISTORY

A 52-year-old female has left eye proptosis and visual deficit.

FINDINGS

Axial and coronal T1-weighted images demonstrate significant proptosis of the left eye. A well-circumscribed, slightly hypointense mass is noted in the medioinferior aspect of the left retrobulbar region with displacement of the left optic nerve laterally and superiorly (Figs. 49.1, 49.2). The mass is predominantly homogeneously hyperintense on T2-weighted image (Fig. 49.3). Postcontrast coronal T1-weighted image reveals intense contrast enhancement. Susceptibility artifact within the globes is from scleral banding.

DIAGNOSIS

Cavernous hemangioma of the left orbit.

DISCUSSION

Cavernous hemangiomas represent 12% to 15% of all adult orbital masses and are the most common adult orbital vascular tumor. Patients often present in the second to the fourth decades of life, with incidence in females being more common.

Cavernous hemangiomas usually follow a characteristic clinical course with slowly progressive tumor enlargement, as opposed to capillary hemangiomas, which gradually diminish in size. Symptoms are related to the tumor mass effect, displacement, or compression of orbital structures, with gradually progressive unilateral proptosis, diplopia, and diminished visual acuity.

Cavernous hemangiomas are usually single and unilateral. They may be located anywhere in the orbit but approximately 83% occur in the retrobulbar muscle cone. Macroscopically, they are well-circumscribed, purplish red lesions with a distinct fibrous pseudocapsule. In contrast to capillary hemangiomas, a prominent arterial supply is usually absent. Rarely, phleboliths may be seen. Histologic characteristic features of the lesions include numerous dilated vascular channels lined by thin, attenuated endothelial cells, often separated by fibrous septa.

On CT, cavernous hemangiomas are well-defined, smoothly marginated, round, ovoid or lobulated, homogeneously hyperdense soft tissue masses with variable contrast enhancement. Unless they are ruptured or surgically violated, cavernous hemangiomas always respect the contour of the globe. Orbital bone remodeling and calcification may sometime be seen.

On MRI, cavernous hemangiomas are usually hyperintense to muscles but hypointense to fat on T1-weighted imaging. Because of the high fluid content in the numerous dilated vascular channels, the tumors are more intense than any other orbital tissues on T2-weighted images. Cavernous hemangiomas usually demonstrate moderately diffuse contrast enhancement. At times, cavernous hemangiomas may be difficult to differentiate from other intraconal lesions such as meningiomas, schwannomas, and hemangiopericytomas. However, in the appropriate clinical setting, the diagnosis is highly suggestive if progressive contrast filling of the tumor is a feature. Uncommonly, an intramuscular hemangioma may occur.

Surgical resection is the treatment of choice. Because the tumors are well-defined, encapsulated, and independent of the general circulation, total excision can usually be accomplished. However, even after an incomplete removal, cavernous hemangiomas usually follow a long period of very slow growth, then a shorter interval of arrest and eventually involution.

SUGGESTED READINGS

Bilaniuk LT, Rapoport RJ. Magnetic resonance imaging of the orbit. *Top Magn Reson Imaging* 1994;6:167–181.

Forbes G. Vascular lesions of the orbit. *Neuroimag Clin North Am* 1996;6:113–222.

Mafee MF, Putterman A, Valvassori GE, et al. Orbital space-occupying lesions: role of CT and MRI. Analysis of 145 cases. *Radiol Clin North Am* 1987;25:529–559.

Mukherji SK, Tart RP, Fitzsimmons J, et al. Fat-suppressed MR of the orbit and cavernous sinus: comparison of fast spin-echo and conventional spin-echo. *AJNR Am J Neuroradiol* 1994;15:1707–1714.

Thorn-Kany M, Arruae P, Delisle MB, et al. Cavernous hemangiomas of the orbit: MR imaging. *J Neuroradiol* 1999;26:79–86.

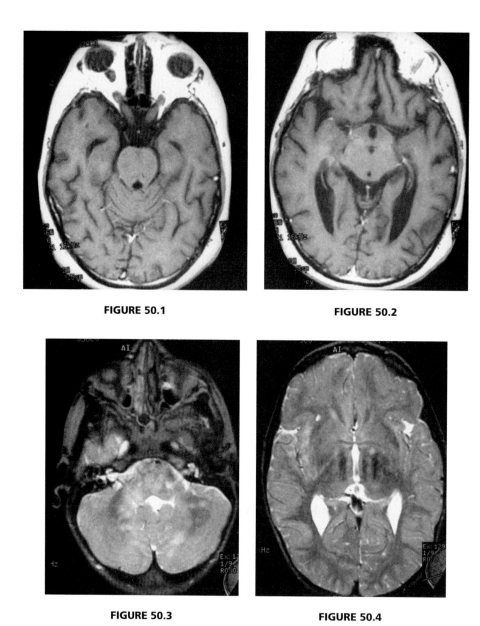

FIGURE 50.1

FIGURE 50.2

FIGURE 50.3

FIGURE 50.4

CLINICAL HISTORY

A 10-year-old boy has a history of multiple skin lesions.

FINDINGS

Contrast-enhanced T1-weighted axial images through the orbit demonstrate enlargement of bilateral optic nerves (Fig. 50.1). No contrast enhancement is seen. The optic chiasm and proximal optic tract is also enlarged, associated with mild compression upon the cerebral peduncle (Fig. 50.2). T2-weighted axial image through the brainstem shows extensive areas of increased signal in the medulla and the middle cerebellar peduncle bilaterally (Fig. 50.3). Similarly, a focal T2 high signal is present in the left lentiform nucleus near the genu of internal capsule and subcortical white matter of the frontal lobe (Fig. 50.4).

DIAGNOSIS

Neurofibromatosis I with bilateral visual apparatus glioma.

DISCUSSION

Neurofibromatosis type 1 (NF1) is the most common among all the phakomatoses. The incidence of NF1 is reported to be 1 in 2,000 to 3,000 live births. NF1 is an autosomal dominant disease transmitted on the long arm of chromosome 17. Diagnosis of NF1 is made when a patient has two or more of the following findings:

1. Six or more café-au-lait spots larger than 5 mm
2. Two or more Lisch nodules (pigmented iris hamartomas)
3. One plexiform neurofibroma or two or more neurofibromas of any type
4. Optic pathway glioma
5. Axillary or inguinal freckling
6. Characteristic skeletal findings (e.g., dysplasia of the greater sphenoid wing, pseudoarthrosis, bowing of the tibia, ribbon ribs, lateral thoracic meningocele, dural ectasia)
7. First degree relative with NF1

Central nervous system (CNS) lesions are seen in 15% to 20% of all patients with NF1. In a patient with NF1, the incidence of developing a CNS neoplasm is 4 times higher than in the general population. The neoplasms associated with NF1 are typically tumors of neurons and astrocytes, unlike lesions associated with NF2, which are tumors of Schwann cells and meninges. Low-grade astrocytomas in brainstem are also seen with increased incidence in NF1.

The common CNS tumor in NF1 is optic nerve glioma, occurring in 5% to 15% of cases, and 25% of all patients with optic gliomas have NF1. Most of optic gliomas are benign low-grade gliomas, usually pilocytic astrocytoma. Optic nerve gliomas can extend into the chiasm, optic tract, lateral geniculate ganglion, and, less commonly, optic radiations. The lesions are hypointense on T1-weighted image and hyperintense on T2-weighted image. Contrast enhancement is variable, but usually minimum to mild in most cases.

Plexiform neurofibromas are a hallmark of NF1 and are infiltrative fusiform unencapsulated masses along major nerves. Plexiform neurofibroma of the first division of the trigeminal nerve is usually associated with dysplasia of the sphenoid wing and buphthalmos.

Hamartomatous lesions in brain are fairly common in NF1 and are seen in 80% of all patients with NF1. These benign nongliomatous lesions are seen in the basal ganglia (particularly globus paladi), brainstem, cerebellum, internal capsule, and centrum semiovale, and they do not show contrast enhancement, edema, or mass effect. Presence of enhancement of these lesions raises the possibility of developing glioma. However, enhancing hypothalamic masses may spontaneously revolve. Therefore, careful clinical follow-up with conservative management is warranted unless increasing mass effect causes symptoms.

The other manifestations of NF1 include intracranial aneurysm and, more commonly, progressive arterial occlusive disease. Spinal cord (intramedullary) lesions are typically low-grade astrocytoma or hamartomatous lesions. Neurofibromas of cranial or peripheral nerve are also seen.

SUGGESTED READINGS

Bognanno JR, Edward MK, Lee TA, et al. Cranial MR imaging in neurofibromatosis. *AJR Am J Roentgenol* 1988;15:381–388.

DiPaolo DP, Zimmerman RA, Rorke LB, et al. Neurofibromatosis type 1: pathologic substrate of high signal intensity foci in the brain. *Radiology* 1995;195:721–724.

Terada H, Barkovich AJ, Edwards MSB, et al. Evaluation of high signal intensity basal ganglia lesions on T1 weighted MR in neurofibromatosis type 1. *AJR Am J Roentgenol* 1996;17:755–760.

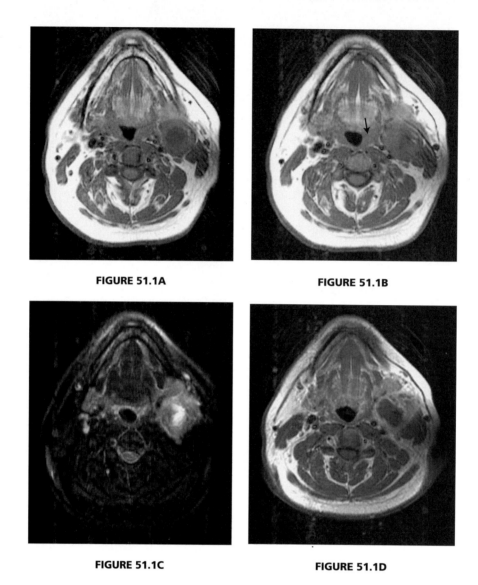

FIGURE 51.1A

FIGURE 51.1B

FIGURE 51.1C

FIGURE 51.1D

CLINICAL HISTORY

A man presents with a mass in the left upper neck.

FINDINGS

A large level IIa (jugulodigastric) node with central areas of noncontrast enhancement on the T1-weighted axial images (Fig. 51.1A, B, D) and high signal intensity on T2-weighted images suggest necrosis (Fig. 51.1C). There is very slight enlargement of the left palatine tonsil. There is no evidence of invasion of the tongue base, mandible, or carotid artery.

DIAGNOSIS

Carcinoma of the left tonsillar fossa with a large level IIa necrotic lymph node.

DISCUSSION

Cancers of the oral cavity and oropharynx are expected to be accessible to inspection or palpation, and thus diagnosed and treated early. However, it is not uncommon for tumors to spread deeply beneath the intact mucosa to other areas of the neck and the skull base that are beyond the limits of physical examination. Imaging plays a significant role in further evaluating the extent of these lesions.

The palatine tonsil lies between the anterior and posterior tonsillar pillars and is the only component of Waldeyer's ring that has a capsule. The capsule is a specialized portion of the pharyngobasilar fascia and separates the tonsil from the superior constrictor muscle.

Carcinoma arising from the tonsillar fossa spreads deeply through the superior constrictor muscle and its fascia to the parapharyngeal space. These tumors commonly spread superiorly to the soft palate along the palatoglossus muscle or nasopharynx via the levator veli palatini muscle. Caudal extension may involve the retromolar trigone and mandibular destruction. Posterior extension may be to the base of tongue and posterior pharyngeal wall. The jugulodigastric lymph node, which is also referred to as the tonsillar node, and deep internal jugular chain are frequently involved.

Diagnosis of tumor involvement in the mandible is important because advanced tumor extending into the mandible is rarely curable with radiation therapy alone. Such significant tumor mass should be managed by surgery or combined therapy. MRI has a great advantage in evaluating marrow involvement with tumor in this area. However, it is difficult to diagnose cortex involvement of the mandible.

Early stage squamous cell carcinoma of the tonsil is amenable to treatment by either surgery or radiation therapy as a single modality, with comparable rates of local control. Unfortunately, manifestation of the disease at an early stage is infrequent. Advanced disease requires treatment with the combination of both surgery and radiation.

SUGGESTED READINGS

Bradford CR, Futran N, Peters G. Management of tonsil cancer. *Head Neck* 1999;21:657–662.

Wang MB, Kuber N, Kerner MM, et al. Tonsillar carcinoma: analysis of treatment results. *J Otolaryngol* 1998;27:263–269.

Yousem DM, Chalian AA. Oral cavity and pharynx. *Radiol Clin North Am* 1998;36:967–981.

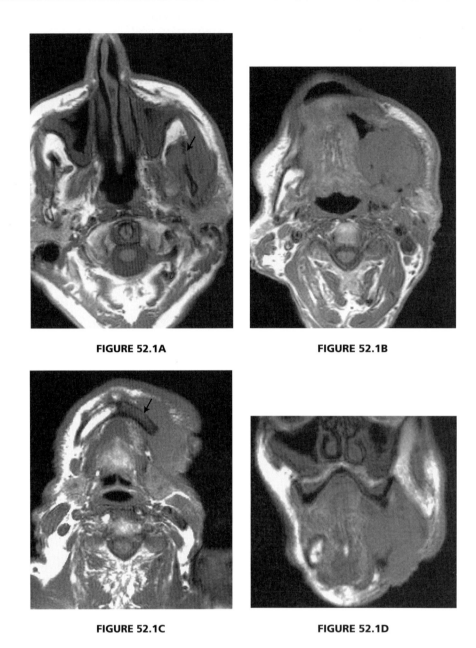

FIGURE 52.1A

FIGURE 52.1B

FIGURE 52.1C

FIGURE 52.1D

CLINICAL HISTORY

A 62-year-old woman has a 40 pack a year history of smoking and occasional alcohol use. Her oral cavity was examined because of multiple complaints.

FINDINGS

T1-weighted axial images show a mass centered in the left masticator space (Fig. 52.1A). Lower sections reveal the main portion of the tumor to be centered in the region of the retromolar trigone (RMT) (Fig. 52.1B). Slightly lower sections show that the mass involves the marrow of the left mandible up to the symphysis (Fig. 52.1C). Coronal images show that there is some invasion of the tongue musculature laterally (Fig. 52.1D).

DIAGNOSIS

Squamous cell carcinoma of the RMT.

DISCUSSION

The oral cavity extends from the skin–vermilion junction of the anterior lips to the junction of the hard and soft palates above and to the line of circumvallate papillae below. It is divided into the following specific areas:

1. Lip
2. Anterior two thirds of tongue
3. Buccal mucosa
4. Floor of mouth
5. Lower gingiva
6. Retromolar trigone
7. Upper gingiva
8. Hard palate

The RMT is the region within the oral cavity best described as the gingiva of the ascending ramus of the mandible. Immediately adjacent to the RMT are the buccal mucosa laterally, the tuberosity of the maxilla and the upper gum superiorly, the floor of the mouth, the faucial arch and soft palate medially, the lower gum anteriorly, and the mandible with the attached muscles of mastication posteriorly. Because of its relatively limited surface area, lesions arising in the RMT frequently invade contiguous structures, resulting in bone invasion and advanced stage.

Squamous cell carcinoma of the RMT is unusual and there is a paucity of information in the world literature describing the radiographic imaging and criteria for selection of treatment. Pain and trismus were the two most frequent complaints. The pain was either in the local area or referred to the ear. According to the study by Byers and colleagues, the most common sites of extension of the cancer in order of frequency were to the tonsillar pillar, lower gingiva, soft palate, and buccal mucosa. The overall incidence of pathologically proven cancer invading bone was 14%. The node most commonly involved in the metastasis was the jugulodigastric.

In almost one third of the patients, another primary cancer developed which was frequently located above the clavicle in the aerodigestive tract. The 5-year survival rate of these patients was 26%. The study suggested that the higher the tumor and node stages, the more likely the patient was selected for surgery as the initial choice of treatment. It showed that every RMT lesion does not require a "commando" type of operation (jaw resection and radical neck dissection) in order to obtain good local-regional control of the cancer.

The presence of extracapsular invasion seems to be an indication for the use of planned combined treatment of surgery and radiotherapy. If there is extensive involvement of the soft palate, the use of radiation may be preferable because surgical resection of the soft palate produces a rather difficult functional deficit for the patient to manage. If there are significant premalignant changes scattered throughout the oral cavity and oropharynx and the patient is a heavy smoker, it might be preferable that surgery be selected as the initial modality of treatment.

The contributions of MRI in RMT lesions are that (a) treatment planning includes evaluation of the status of surrounding deep anatomic structures, which are not accessible clinically, (b) secondary primary lesions can be detected, (c) neck node status can be determined, and (d) mandibular invasion can be detected. In general, MRI of squamous cell carcinoma in oral lesions characteristically shows low to isointense signal on T1-weighted images, bright signal on T2-weighted images, and gadolinium enhancement on T1-weighted images.

SUGGESTED READINGS

Byers RM, et al. Treatment of squamous carcinoma of retromolar trigone. *Am J Clin Oncol* 1984;7:647–652.
Shan JP, et al. The patterns of cervical lymph node metastases: squamous carcinoma of the oral cavity. *Cancer* 1990;66:109–113.

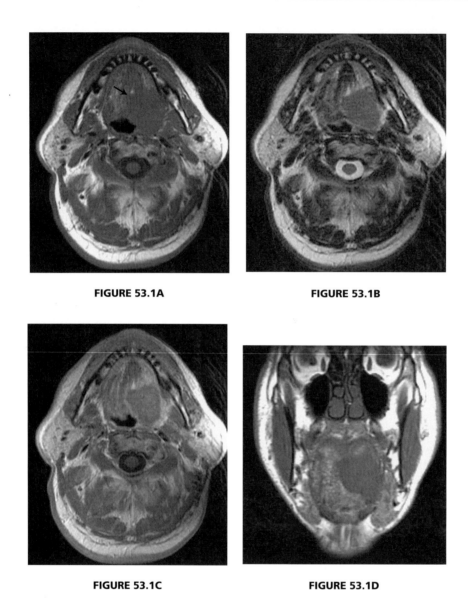

FIGURE 53.1A   FIGURE 53.1B

FIGURE 53.1C   FIGURE 53.1D

CLINICAL HISTORY

A previously healthy 48-year-old man presents with a 3-month history of progressive soreness of the tongue and dysphagia. The patient admitted to a long history of tobacco use (three to four cigars a day).

CLINICAL HISTORY

The axial T1-weighted image shows a mass in the left base of the tongue that extends posteriorly toward the tonsil (Fig. 53.1A). Notice that the tumor appears isointense with the normal musculature of the tongue. The T2-weighted axial image shows increased signal intensity around the periphery of the mass, which is easily distinguished from adjacent muscle (Fig. 53.1B). The contrast-enhanced T1-weighted image adds little information (Fig. 53.1C). The coronal T1-weighted image confirms these findings (Fig. 53.1D). Important observations are that the tumor crosses the midline of the tongue and does not grossly involve the mandible cortex, marrow, or carotid artery.

DIAGNOSIS

Squamous cell carcinoma of the base of the left tongue.

DISCUSSION

Squamous cell carcinoma accounts for more than 90% of malignant neoplasms of the oral cavity and oropharynx. Adenocarcinoma, lymphoma, minor salivary gland malignancies, and other rare neoplasms account for the remaining 10%. The two major risk factors associated with tumors of squamous cell origin in this region of the head and neck have long been recognized and are tobacco and alcohol. Despite the common histology of the tumors, their behavior depends on their location in the mouth. In general, a "malignant gradient" and likelihood of metastases increases with a more posterior location in the oral cavity and pharynx.

Anterior lesions (carcinoma of the lips, buccal mucosa, gingiva, alveolar mucosa, and anterior tongue) are generally moderately to well differentiated and metastasize relatively late to regional nodes (submandibular nodes). They are also relatively easy to evaluate clinically, and, therefore, CT and MR imaging have limited usefulness in this area.

Carcinomas of the floor of the mouth, on the other hand, are usually moderately to poorly differentiated and metastasize early to bilateral regional (submandibular, sublingual, and high jugular) nodes. Tumors of the base of the tongue (posterior one third) tend to be diagnosed at a more advanced stage than tumors of the oral (anterior two thirds) tongue. Tongue base cancers tend to be more aggressive than those of the oral tongue. Their poorer prognosis is also due to overall larger size and increased incidence of nodal metastasis at the time of diagnosis. Approximately 70% of patients with tongue base tumors present with advanced disease (stage III or IV) compared with 30% of patients with carcinomas of the oral tongue. Tongue base cancers may spread laterally to involve the mandible, anteriorly to involve the oral tongue, and inferiorly to involve the preepiglottic space and supraglottic larynx. Lymphatic spread may occur bilaterally to submandibular, sublingual, and high jugular nodes.

The presence of nodal disease affects the staging of tumors, the patient's overall prognosis, and whether a nodal dissection will be performed with the primary surgical resection. High in the neck and deep to the sternocleidomastoid muscle, adenopathy can be inaccessible to palpation and is best evaluated with an imaging study.

When the carotid artery is involved with tumor, the chance for a primary surgical cure is greatly reduced, and the overall treatment of the patient must be reevaluated. MR images can show to what extent the vessel in question is surrounded by tumor. As well, when tumor extends to the mandible, the likelihood of a cure by radiation therapy is greatly reduced, and surgery must be considered. Although the dense cortical bone of the mandible produces no signal on MR images, MRI can still resolve tumor involvement because replacement of the normal low signal of cortical bone is evidence of tumor invasion.

It is often difficult to clinically evaluate the deep floor of mouth and tongue base because deep palpation of this area often causes gagging and is therefore intolerable to most patients. Therefore, CT and especially MRI play an important role in identifying lesions and determining tumor extent. Carcinoma tends to have a low signal intensity (long T1) on T1-weighted images, which makes it difficult to differentiate from normal musculature. On T2-weighted images, the tumor has varying degrees of high signal intensity, which allows sharp differentiation of the tumor from the low intensity surrounding musculature. Normal lymphoid tissue also has increased signal on T2-weighted images that may be confused with tumor. The lack of infiltration helps to separate this benign process. The excellent tissue differentiation and spatial resolution of MRI allow the detection of tumor spread along tissue planes, vascular channels, and muscle bundles.

Because the definite diagnosis of cancer is obtained primarily by biopsy, the role of CT and MRI is to provide an accurate staging workup in planning therapy. It is clinically important to determine whether the tumor has spread over the midline of the lingual septum, to the mandible, and to the pharynx. The determination of sparing or involvement of the lingual artery and hypoglossal nerve predicts the appropriateness of partial or hemiglossectomy.

As the tumors extend slightly further cephalad and anteriorly beneath the horizontal intrinsic muscle plane, they encroach on the two bundles of the genioglossus muscle. Because the main bulk of the tongue is formed by this paired genioglossus muscle, most tumors involve the genioglossus muscle to some extent. The genioglossus is always separated by a midline low-density raphe. If this low-density region is obliterated, it is a reliable sign of infiltration across the midline by a tumor mass.

The two bundles of the genioglossus should be quite symmetrical and their fan-shaped course from caudad to cephalad is also an excellent landmark on coronal and sagittal scanning. Anteriorly and to either side of the genioglossus muscles are broad, low-density planes between it and the mylohyoid muscles. In this groove lie the sublingual salivary glands and the duct of the submandibular gland. Infiltrating lesions of the floor of the mouth or extension of tumor into the mobile tongue will obliterate these low-density planes.

Both surgery and radiation therapy are used for treating lesions in this area.

SUGGESTED READINGS

Arakawa A, Tsuruta J, Nishimura R, et al. Lingual carcinoma. Correlation of MR imaging with histopathological findings. *Acta Radiol* 1996;37:700–707.

Crecco M, Vidiri A, Palma O, et al. T stages of tumors of the tongue and floor of the mouth: correlation between MR with gadopentetate dimeglumine and pathologic data. *Am J Neuroradiol* 1994;15:1695–1702.

Lufkin RB, Wortham DG, Dietrich RB, et al. Tongue and oropharynx: findings on MR imaging. *Radiology* 1986;161:69–75.

Sigal R, Zagdanski AM, Schwaab G, et al. CT and MR imaging of squamous cell carcinoma of the tongue and floor of the mouth. *Radiographics* 1996;16:787–810.

Yasumoto M, Shibuya H, Takeda M, et al. Squamous cell carcinoma of the oral cavity: MR findings and value of T1- versus T2-weighted fast spin-echo images. *AJR Am J Roentgenol* 1995;164:981–987.

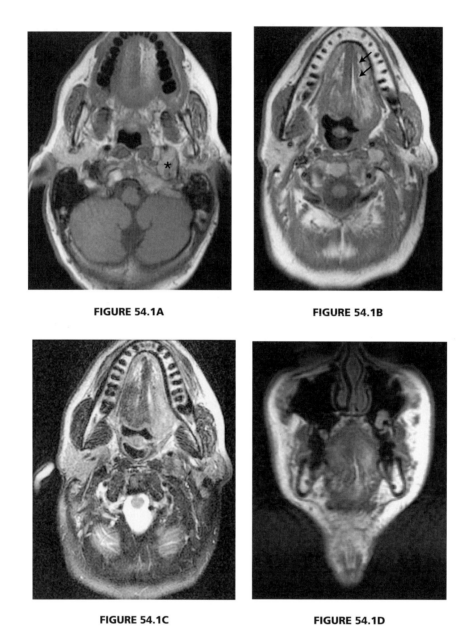

FIGURE 54.1A   **FIGURE 54.1B**

FIGURE 54.1C   **FIGURE 54.1D**

CLINICAL HISTORY

A 45-year-old man was referred for evaluation of a right-sided tongue mass.

FINDINGS

Noncontrast T1-weighted axial images show asymmetrically larger right side of the tongue with increased signal intensity on the left side of the tongue. In addition, there is a skull base mass on the left (Fig. 54.1A). Axial T1-weighted images slightly lower reveal smaller genioglossus muscles on the left (Fig. 54.1B). Axial T2-weighted images confirm these findings (Fig. 54.1C). Coronal images show the fatty replacement of the left hemiglossus (Fig. 54.1D).

DIAGNOSIS

Hypoglossal denervation atrophy.

DISCUSSION

The hypoglossal nerve is the motor nerve of the tongue musculature. The clinical appearance of hypoglossal palsy may range from slight muscle fasciculation in early or mild involvement to obvious atrophy in severe cases. In the acute/subacute phase, there may be muscular edema. Muscular wasting occurs after 2 to 3 weeks in any peripheral lesion to a motor nerve. Permanent damage leads to muscle atrophy and replacement of the muscle fibers by fat and fibrous tissue. Unilateral hypoglossal nerve palsy results in selective atrophy of the intrinsic and extrinsic muscles of the tongue. Flaccidity of the muscles can result in a pseudomass on the side of the lesion.

The hypoglossal nerve leaves the skull base through the hypoglossal canal medially and above the occipital condyle, close to the anterior rim of the foramen magnum. It may be divided into five segments: the medullary, cisternal, skull base, nasopharyngeal/oropharyngeal carotid space, and sublingual segments. Each segment is usually affected by different disorders. Localizing a lesion to a particular segment allows the radiologist to narrow the differential diagnosis.

Beyond the skull base, the hypoglossal nerve is joined by motor nerves from the C1–2 roots of the ansa cervicalis. These cervical branches proceed unmodified to the geniohyoid muscle and do not exchange fibers with the hypoglossal nerve. Therefore, depending on the site of the lesion, the geniohyoid muscle may or may not be spared. The mylohyoid muscles and anterior bellies of the digastric muscles remain unaffected with hypoglossal palsy.

Both CT and MRI are useful in assessing dysfunction of the hypoglossal nerve. Recent denervation results in edema-like attenuation or signal intensity changes and abnormal contrast enhancement in the denervated musculature. One recent study noted no such contrast enhancement in radiation-induced hypoglossal denervation. In this early stage, the base of the ipsilateral side of the tongue appears expanded with increased signal intensity on T2-weighted images. The appearance is characteristic in longstanding denervation with extensive fatty infiltration and atrophy of the affected musculature.

When findings of unilateral muscular fatty infiltration of the tongue are present on CT or MRI, a lesion along the course of the ipsilateral hypoglossal nerve from the tongue to the brainstem should be excluded. In one large series, almost half of the patients presenting with hypoglossal palsy were found to have a malignant tumor as the underlying etiology.

SUGGESTED READINGS

Batchelor TT, Krol GS, DeAngelis LM. Neuroimaging abnormalities with hypoglossal nerve palsies. *J Neuroimaging* 1996;6:240–242.

Keane JR. Twelfth-nerve palsy. Analysis of 100 cases. *Arch Neurol* 1996;53:561–566.

King AD, AhuJa A, Leung SF, et al. MR features of the denervated tongue in radiation induced neuropathy. *Br J Radiol* 1999;72:349–353.

Russo CP, Smoker WR, Weissman JL. MR appearance of the trigeminal and hypoglossal motor denervation. *AJNR Am J Neuroradiol* 1997;18:1375–1383.

Thompson EO, Smoker WR. Hypoglossal nerve palsy: a segmental approach. *Radiographics* 1994;14:939–958.

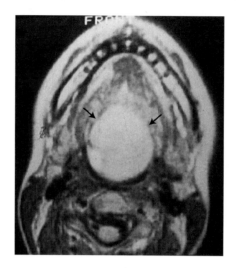

FIGURE 55.1A

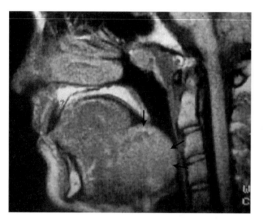

FIGURE 55.1B

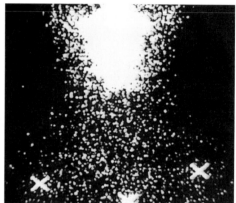

FIGURE 55.1C

CLINICAL HISTORY

An adult woman presents with a long history of a swelling of the floor of the mouth.

FINDINGS

An axial T1-weighted image shows a rounded, well-defined 3 × 3 cm heterogeneous mass in the central posterior tongue (Fig. 55.1A). Note that the mass is in the midline of the tongue and is at the posterior third of that structure. The mass shows a slightly higher T1-weighted signal intensity compared with the normal muscles of the tongue on both axial and sagittal views (Fig. 55.1B). The mass displaces the free margin of the epiglottis posteriorly but does not invade that structure. The radiolabeled iodine (^{131}I) study shows activity within the mass and no activity in the normal thyroid bed (Fig. 55.1C). (Images courtesy of Dr. Thomas Vogl.)

DIAGNOSIS

Lingual thyroid.

DISCUSSION

The primordial thyroid forms an epithelial lined tube known as the thyroglossal duct (see Case 29 and Case 36). The embryologic thyroid tissue arises within the foramen cecum (behind the circum vallate papillae of the tongue) and descends along the hyoid bone to the thyroid isthmus. The thyroid gland normally traverses the length of the thyroglossal duct to reach its final position anterolateral to the trachea.

This migration may be arrested at any point. When the thyroid fails to migrate below the tongue it is known as a lingual thyroid. Even with a normal appearing thyroid gland, residual thyroid tissue may appear anywhere along the thyroglossal duct. The reported incidence of ectopic tissue along the tract varies from 0.5% to 35.0%.

Patients may present with an asymptomatic posterior reddish tongue base mass. The incidence of lingual thyroid is slightly higher in women than men.

On MRI, the lingual thyroid appears as a relatively homogeneous mass at midline below the foramen cecum. On CT scanning, the ectopic thyroid has the same x-ray increased attenuation features (due to intrinsic iodine) found in normally located thyroid tissue. Radiolabeled iodine may be used to define the location of the active thyroid tissue. If surgery is contemplated, a radiolabeled iodine scan is often performed to confirm the presence of other normally functioning tissue elsewhere in the neck.

All of the pathologic conditions, both benign and malignant, that may be found in normally located thyroid tissue may also occur in ectopic thyroid.

SUGGESTED READINGS

Douglas PS, Baker AW. Lingual thyroid. *Br J Oral Maxillofac Surg* 1994;32:123–124.

Giovagnorio F, Cordier A, Romeo R. Lingual thyroid: value of integrated imaging. *Eur Radiol* 1996;6:105–107.

Hsu CY, Wang SJ. Thyroid hemiagenesis accompanying an ectopic sublingual thyroid. *Clin Nucl Med* 1994;19:546.

Jayaram G, Kakar A, Prakash R. Papillary carcinoma arising in sublingual ectopic thyroid concentrating both Tc-99m pertechnetate and I-131. Diagnosis by fine needle aspiration cytology. *Clin Nucl Med* 1995;20:381–383.

Vogl T, Brüning R, Grevers G, et al. MR Imaging of the oropharynx and tongue: comparison of plain and Gd-DTPA studies. *J Comput Assist Tomogr* 1988;12:427–433.

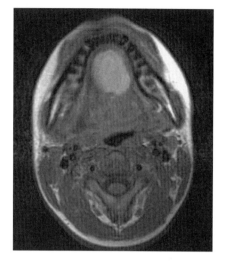

FIGURE 56.1A

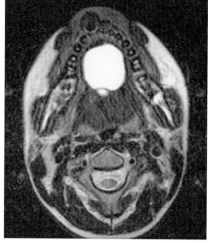

FIGURE 56.1B

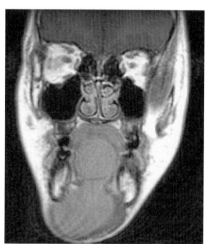

FIGURE 56.1C

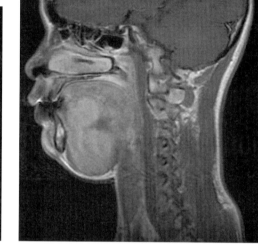

FIGURE 56.1D

CLINICAL HISTORY

A 26-year-old man has a long-term history of a swelling in the floor of the mouth.

FINDINGS

A well-defined midline floor of the mouth mass that is hyperintense relative to muscle on axial T1-weighted images is found (Fig. 56.1A). On T2-weighted image, it is very high signal (Fig. 56.1B). The coronal image shows the mass to be located between the genioglossus muscles and to extend below the mandible (Fig. 56.1C). The increased signal on T1-weighted images may be due to a combination of lipid content and complex proteinaceous fluid. The sagittal MRI confirms these findings (Fig. 56.1D).

DIAGNOSIS

Epidermoid or "dermoid" cyst of the floor of the mouth (sublingual).

DISCUSSION

Dermoid cysts are epithelial lined cavities with associated skin appendages, including hair, hair follicles, and sebaceous glands. The epithelial tissue usually arises from embryonic rests and occasionally from traumatic or iatrogenic implantation. Of dermoid cysts of the head and neck, 25% occur in the oral cavity, usually in the anterior floor of the mouth.

The term "dermoid cyst" is used to describe several histologically distinct types of cysts in the head and neck. Most are localized to the orbit, oral cavity, and sinonasal regions. The more common epidermoid cysts are lined with simple squamous cell epithelium and contain no skin appendage. Rare teratoid cysts contain derivatives of skin appendages, endoderm, and mesoderm. All three types of cysts may contain a cheesy keratinaceous material.

Dermoid cysts of the oral cavity usually present in the midline anterior floor of the mouth in the second or third decade of life. Such cysts may be either acquired implantations or congenital enclaves of tissue and are subclassified into sublingual and submental varieties.

Sublingual dermoids are superior to the mylohyoid muscle, splitting the midline extrinsic tongue muscles (geniohyoid–genioglossus complex) to occupy the floor of the mouth. Less frequently, the sublingual cyst may be laterally located, displacing the geniohyoid complex medially.

Submental dermoids lie inferior to the mylohyoid muscle, between it and the platysma, and tend to present as an anterior neck mass. Either type may elevate the tongue, interfere with deglutition, or grow to a large size and present as a submandibular mass.

These lesions are invariably midline and may be found either above the mylohyoid in the sublingual space or below it in the submental space. Sublingual dermoids may raise the tongue and simulate a ranula. Submental space dermoids present as a neck mass.

Dermoids tend to lie anterior to the foramen cecum region (which makes a thyroglossal duct cyst less likely). They are generally well circumscribed. Dermoid cysts may contain various amounts of hair, calcification, fluid, or fat.

Dermoid tumors are typically hyperintense on T1- and T2-weighted images as a result of the short T1 and intermediate T2 caused by the high lipid content within the cyst. Other tumors have demonstrated variable degrees of T1 and T2 lengthening, related to a variety of contained elements, or areas of signal void if regions of dense focal calcification are present. Tumors rich in keratin debris have long T1 and T2 signal intensities, whereas tumors rich in cholesterin (lipid) have short T1 signal intensities that fade on T2-weighted images. Some cysts may show a characteristic fluid level on MR. If a portion of the fluid within dermoid cysts is rich in lipids, a chemical shift artifact is generated in the direction of the frequency-encoding gradient.

On CT, dermoid cysts appear as round, well-circumscribed, low-density masses that may appear multiloculated or contain fat and calcific densities as well as fluid.

SUGGESTED READINGS

Batsakis JG. *Tumors of the head and neck: clinical and pathological considerations,* 2nd ed. Baltimore: Williams and Wilkins, 1979;226–228.

Davidson HD, Ouchi T, Steiner RE. NMR imaging of congenital intracranial germinal layer neoplasms. *Neuroradiology* 1985;27:301–303.

Dillon WP, Miller EM. Cervical soft tissues. In: Newton TH, Hasso AN, Dillon WP, ed. *Modern neuroradiology, vol. 3. Computed tomography of the head and neck.* New York: Raven Press, 1988;11.31–11.33.

Hunter TB, Palplanus SH, Chernin MM, et al. Dermoid cyst of the floor of the mouth: CT appearance. *AJR Am J Roentgenol* 1983;141:1239–1240.

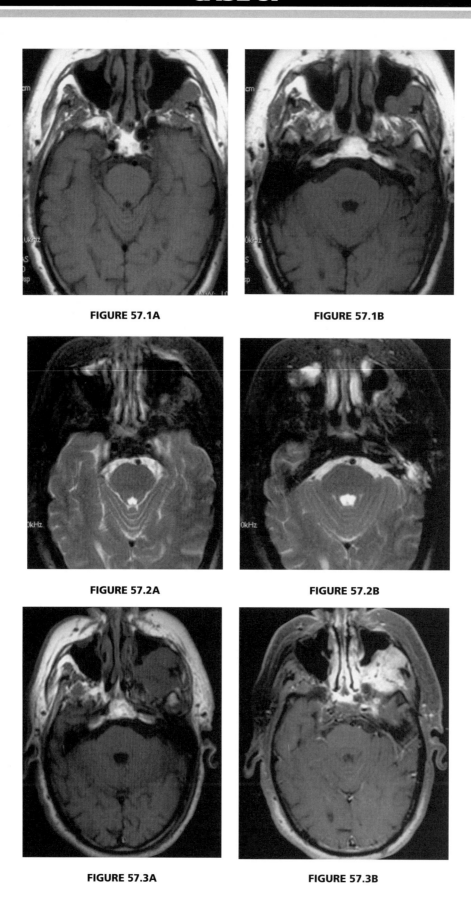

FIGURE 57.1A

FIGURE 57.1B

FIGURE 57.2A

FIGURE 57.2B

FIGURE 57.3A

FIGURE 57.3B

CLINICAL HISTORY

A 68-year-old man with history of squamous cell carcinoma of the hard palate is treated with surgery and radiation therapy. He undergoes a routine follow-up MR examination.

FINDINGS

T1-weighted images show a focal nodular soft tissue in the anterior left masticator space with obliteration of the retroantral fat pad (Fig. 57.1A, B). On T2-weighted image, the lesion is low in signal and more inconspicuous than that on T1-weighted image (Fig. 57.2A, B). The abnormality was not detected as a potential recurrent tumor.

Six months later, precontrast and postcontrast T1-weighted images show extensive tumor recurrence in the skull base (Fig. 57.3A, B).

DIAGNOSIS

Recurrent squamous cell carcinoma of the palate.

DISCUSSION

Approximately 90% of oral cavity malignant tumors are squamous cell carcinoma. Other malignant tumors in this region include minor salivary gland tumor (adenoid cystic carcinoma, adenocarcinoma, mucoepidermoid carcinoma), lymphoma, and rare sarcoma. The primary roles of imaging study for squamous cell carcinoma of the oral cavity are to define the extent of a primary tumor and to assess the status of cervical lymph node metastasis. For the hard palate carcinoma, special attention should be paid to involvement of the mandible, floor of the maxillary sinus and nasal cavity, and soft palate, as well as presence of perineural extension.

Interpretation of MRI of the postoperative head and neck cancer can be challenging. It is important to carefully search for any mass or nodular soft tissue to indicate recurrent tumor. Noncontrast T1-weighted image provides the basic anatomic information with high contrast between recurrent tumor and adjacent fat. Obliteration of normal fat with nodular soft tissue should raise the possibility of recurrent tumor and requires clinical correlation or biopsy. Ill-defined areas of signal change without a mass effect could be due to prior surgery; therefore, comparison with a baseline postoperative imaging study is valuable. High signal on T2-weighted image is not always reliable in the extracranial head and neck for cancer detection, because many head and neck cancers of the upper aerodigestive tract are often isointense to slightly low signal on T2-weighted image. Contrast enhanced image with fat suppression is also helpful to detect a recurrent head and neck neoplasm and evaluation of perineural spread of tumor and dural extension.

Once a recurrent tumor involves the skull base, pterygopalatine fossa, or foramen rotundum, the prognosis is dismal. The primary goal of postoperative follow-up imaging study is to find a subclinical recurrent tumor, or at least a suspicious area to aid biopsy, so that early and effective treatment is administered.

SUGGESTED READINGS

Lufkin R, Wortham DG, Dietrich RB, et al. Tongue and oropharynx: findings on MR imaging. *Radiology* 1986;161:69–75.
Mukherji SK, Weissman JL, Holiday RA. Upper aerodigestive tract. In Som PM, Curtin HD, eds. *Head and Neck Imaging,* 3rd ed. St. Louis: Mosby, 1996;437–487.

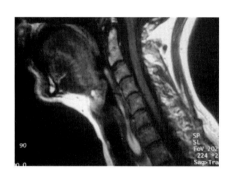

FIGURE 58.1A

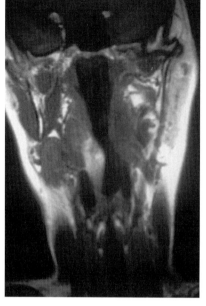

FIGURE 58.1B

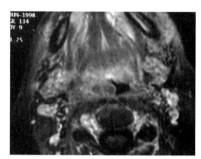

FIGURE 58.1C

CLINICAL HISTORY

The patient is a 49-year-old woman with a longstanding history of mild dyspnea and recent onset of occasional difficulty swallowing.

FINDINGS

Sagittal and coronal T1-weighted and axial postcontrast fat saturated images show a polypoid, pedunculated soft tissue mass arising in the region of the right pallatine tonsil and extending inferiorly, along the posterior wall of the hypopharynx, into the proximal cervical esophagus. The mass has a hyperintense core on T1-weighted images, which enhances after contrast.

DIAGNOSIS

Giant fibrovascular polyp of the oropharynx.

DISCUSSION

Fibrovascular polyps are benign submucosal lesions most commonly arising from the esophagus and hypopharynx; 85% to 90% occur in the vicinity of the cricopharyngeal muscle. They are thought to originate from nodular submucosal thickenings or redundant submucosal folds, which, because of an increase in intrinsic mucosal tension associated with lack of muscular support, evaginate into the surrounding connective tissues. Then, through a mechanism of traction triggered by peristaltic activity, the size of these evaginations progressively increase. Two areas of decreased resistance have been described in the pharyngeal wall: one between the superior and inferior cricopharyngeal muscles (Killian's dehiscence) and the other between the cricopharyngeal muscle and the proximal end of the esophagus

(Laimer's triangle). However, it is thought that small submucosal lesions subject to pressure changes associated with deglutition may be pushed and evaginate toward the pharyngeal lumen.

Pathologically, these polyps are mainly composed of a mixture of fibrous elements, adipose tissue, and vessels. Depending on the preponderant elements, they may be subdivided into fibromas, fibrolipomas, and fibrovascular polyps. Clinical findings range from vague prolonged symptoms to life-threatening episodes of asphyxiation caused by airway obstruction. Because these polyps partially fill the pharynx and may obstruct the laryngeal airway, dysphagia, dysphonia, odynophagia, and episodes of choking sensation are the most commonly reported symptoms. After an episode of coughing or eructation, polyps may be regurgitated.

Diagnosis is difficult in that, on endoscopy, the mucosal lining of the polyp may be mistaken for normal pharyngeal or esophageal mucosa. Cross-sectional imaging is very helpful not only to detect these masses but also to determine their site of origin and extent. Because of its multiplanar capability and high soft tissue resolution, MR is the modality best suited for these purposes. Fibrovascular polyps manifest as pedunculated, smoothly marginated, submucosal masses made up of a stalk and a more globular distal ending (Fig. 58.1A). The imaging features depend on tissue composition.

Fatty elements appear hyperintense on T1-weighted image and of intermediate intensity on T2-weighted images; fibrous components are hypointense on both the T1- and T2-weighted images, and, finally, the vascular elements are responsible for lesion enhancement.

Once the diagnosis is made, these tumors should be managed surgically using laser or cryocoagulation to avoid airway obstruction and asphyxiation.

SUGGESTED READINGS

Le Blanc J, Carrier G, Ferland S, et al. Fibrovascular polyp of the esophagus with computed tomographic and pathologic correlation. *Can Assoc Radiol J* 1990;87–89.

Lee KN, Auh JY, Nam KJ, et al. Regurgitated fibrovascular polyp of the esophagus (letter). *AJR Am J Roentgenol* 1996;166:730.

Owens JJ, Donovan DT, Alford EL, et al. Life threatening presentations of fibrovascular esophageal and hypopharyngeal polyps. *Ann Otol Rhinol Laryngol* 1994;103:838–842.

Walters NA, Coral A. Fibrovascular polyp of the esophagus. The appearances on computed tomography. *Br J Radiol* 1988;61:641–643.

Whitman GJ, Borkowski GP. Giant fibrovascular polyp of the esophagus. *AJR Am J Roentgenol* 1989;152:518–520.

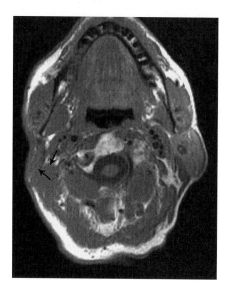

FIGURE 59.1A

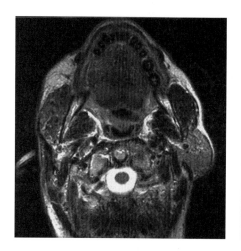

FIGURE 59.1B

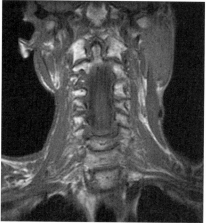

FIGURE 59.1C

CLINICAL HISTORY

A woman presents with facial asymmetry and excessive sweating over the cheek area with meals.

FINDINGS

Axial and coronal T1-weighted images and axial T2-weighted images show an asymmetrically small right parotid gland (Fig. 59.1A, B). The remainder of the surrounding structures are unremarkable.

DIAGNOSIS

Normal postoperative findings following total parotidectomy.

DISCUSSION

Asymmetry of the parotid gland can be due to a number of conditions. Postobstructive and postradiation atrophy can result in a small gland; however, complete absence with these conditions is uncommon. A total parotidectomy leaves little normal glandular tissue whereas a superficial parotidectomy leaves the portion of the gland deep to the plane of the facial nerve (deep lobe of the gland). Gustatory sweating is a well-known sequela of parotid surgery.

Gustatory sweating is also known as Frey (auriculotemporal nerve) syndrome. In this interesting condition, the secretory parasympathetic fibers of the parotid gland are thought to communicate with the sympathetic nerve fibers of sweat glands and blood vessels of the skin following parotidectomy. Miscommunication results in gustatory sweating and facial flushing, which appear early with mastication in the postoperative period.

The diagnosis of postoperative changes can be made by the patient history but should also be recognizable from the imaging findings. Patients with Frey syndrome have facial flushing, sweating, or both localized to the distribution of the auriculotemporal nerve that occurs in response to gustatory stimuli. Up to 40% of patients in some series report this condition following parotid surgery or trauma. It has also been reported as a rare complication of diabetes.

Either MRI or CT can show the soft tissue anatomy of this area well. If there is a question of calculi, CT is the preferred study. Postobstructive or postradiation atrophy may show alteration of signal intensity as well as volume loss of the gland. If the patient's surgical history is unclear or absent, the radiologist should be able to suggest the correct diagnosis.

SUGGESTED READINGS

Yamashita T, Tomoda K, Kumazawa T. The usefulness of partial parotidectomy for benign parotid gland tumors. A retrospective study of 306 cases. *Acta Otolaryngol Suppl* 1993;500:113–116.

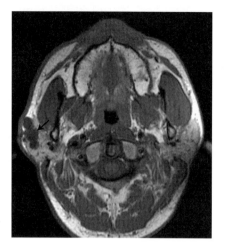

FIGURE 60.1A

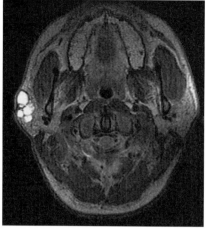

FIGURE 60.1B

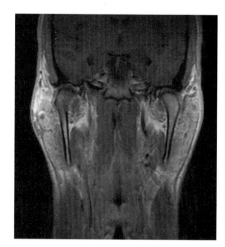

FIGURE 60.1C

CLINICAL HISTORY

A 35-year-old patient with a painless left cheek mass.

FINDINGS

A relatively homogeneous multilobulated mass is noted in the superficial lobe of the left parotid gland (Fig. 60.1A). The lesion is hyperintense on T2-weighted axial images (Fig. 60.1B). On the coronal postcontrast T1-weighted image, there is heterogeneous enhancement and the lesion becomes nearly isointense with the surrounding gland (Fig. 60.1C).

DIAGNOSIS

Pleomorphic adenoma (benign mixed tumor).

DISCUSSION

Salivary gland tumors affect 1 to 3 persons in every 100,000 individuals. Approximately 70% of parotid, 50% of submandibular, 30% of sublingual, and 10% to 40% of accessory salivary gland tumors are benign. It appears that the smaller the salivary gland of origin, the less likely that the tumor is benign.

Pleomorphic adenoma (or benign mixed tumor) is the most common benign salivary gland tumor and the most common tumor of the parotid gland, accounting for 65% of all parotid gland neoplasms. Pleomorphic adenoma occurs in all age groups, although 60% occurs between the third and fifth decades of life with the female to male ratio of more than 2:1. Pleomorphic adenomas tend to be solitary lesions with true multicentric origin being rare.

Pleomorphic adenomas are typically slow-growing painless masses varying greatly in size, from a few millimeters to several centimeters. The tumor is composed of a combination of myoepithelial cells and a variety of epithelial and mesenchymal tissue surrounded by a fibrous capsule. Although it is well encapsulated, it is not uncommon for small areas of neoplastic cells to extend beyond the capsule, known as *satellitosis*. Simple surgical enucleation may leave these areas behind, resulting in residual disease.

Untreated pleomorphic adenomas may undergo malignant transformation in 1% to 25% of cases, mostly in the form of carcinoma ex-pleomorphic adenoma. This should be suspected in patients with longstanding tumors that show a sudden increase in size or development of new symptoms, especially pain and facial nerve paralysis.

On CT, most pleomorphic adenomas are smoothly marginated, spherical lesions of higher attenuation than the surrounding parotid gland. The smaller tumors are usually homogeneous whereas the larger ones are often heterogeneous as a result of areas of necrosis, hemorrhage, and cystic changes. No significant contrast enhancement is expected. Dystrophic calcification, although uncommonly seen, does suggest the diagnosis of pleomorphic adenoma, because this finding is unusual in other parotid tumors.

On MRI, pleomorphic adenomas are usually intermediate on T1-weighted and intermediate to high signal intensity on T2-weighted images. MR characteristics that may suggest malignancy include irregular margination, heterogeneous signal, lymphadenopathy, adjacent soft tissue or bony invasion, and facial perineural spread.

Approximately 10% of parotid pleomorphic adenomas are in the deep lobe. The deep lobe of the parotid gland is the portion of the gland that is deep to the plane of the facial nerve. In true deep lobe tumors, there is absence of the fatty tissue plane, on some or all axial images, between the parapharyngeal deep lobe mass and the normal parotid gland. Normal parotid tissue partially wraps around the lesion, or extension of the lesion laterally into the stylomandibular tunnel further suggests a deep parotid lobe origin. Deep lobe tumors may extend to the prestyloid compartment of the parapharyngeal space, displacing the internal carotid artery posteriorly. Because of different surgical planning (transparotid versus transcervical, transoral, or a combination of these), it is imperative that masses arising from the deep lobe be differentiated from other parapharyngeal space masses.

Surgery, whether superficial or a total parotidectomy, is the treatment of choice for all parotid pleomorphic adenomas. Simple excision is generally not done because of the risk of residual disease.

SUGGESTED READINGS

Curtin HD. Assessment of salivary gland pathology. *Otolaryngol Clin North Am* 1988;21:547–573.

Murphy RJ, Hendrix JD. Unusual presentation of a salivary pleomorphic adenoma: a case report and review of the literature. *Cutis* 1999;63:167–168.

Som PM, Shugar JM, Sacher M, et al. Benign and malignant parotid pleomorphic adenomas: CT and MR studies. *J Comput Assist Tomogr* 1988;25:65–69.

Som PM, Biller HF. High grade malignancies of the parotid gland: identification with MR imaging. *Radiology* 1989;173:823–826.

Som PM, Braun IF, Shapiro MD, et al. Tumors of the parapharyngeal space and upper neck: MR imaging characteristics. *Radiology* 1987;164:823–829.

Swartz JD, Rothman MI, Marlowe FI, et al. MR imaging of parotid mass lesions: attempts at histopathologic differentiation. *J Comput Assist Tomogr* 1989;13:789–796.

Tabor EK, Curtin HD. MR of the salivary glands. *Radiol Clin North Am* 1989;27:379–392.

Teresi LM, Lufkin RB, Wortham DG, et al. Parotid masses: MR imaging. *Radiology* 1987;163:405–409.

Uslu SS, Inal E, Ataoglu O, et al. Pleomorphic adenoma of an unusual size in the deep lobe of the parotid gland. *Int J Pediatr Otorhinolaryngol* 1995;33:163–191.

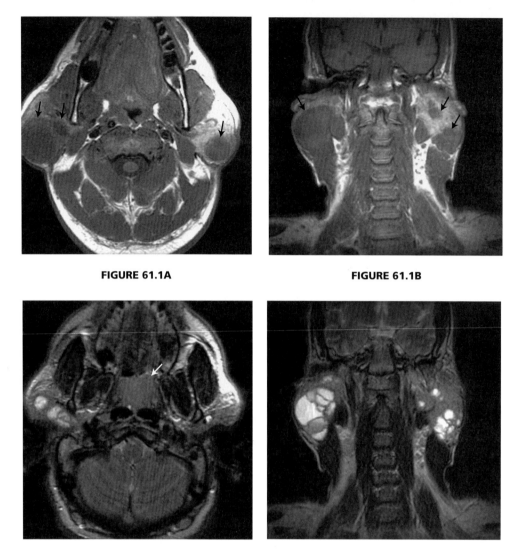

FIGURE 61.1A

FIGURE 61.1B

FIGURE 61.1C

FIGURE 61.1D

CLINICAL HISTORY

A 35-year-old woman has bilateral parotid fullness. Her husband is human immunodeficiency virus positive (HIV+).

FINDINGS

T1-weighted images reveal multiple bilateral intraparotid masses (Fig. 61.1A, B). On the T2-weighted images, they appear to have thin walls and are cystic (Fig. 61.1C, D). No discrete solid parotid masses are present. The higher axial T2-weighted images show extensive adenoidal lymphoid tissue (Fig. 61.1C).

DIAGNOSIS

HIV-associated benign lymphoepithelial cysts.

DISCUSSION

Isolated benign lymphoepithelial cysts (BLC) is a rare disorder of the parotid gland with a reported incidence of 0.6% in the general population. However, there is a strong association (92%) of BLC with HIV+ and patients with acquired immunodeficiency syndrome (AIDS) in whom the incidence of multiple and bilateral parotid lymphoepithelial cysts is 3% to 10%. Interestingly, parotid lymphoepithelial cysts may manifest before HIV seroconversion.

The cysts are typically located in the superficial portion of the parotid gland. Most are bilateral and epithelial lined. The etiology of these cysts remains unclear. The hypothesis of the development of HIV-associated lymphoepithelial cysts from preexisting salivary lymph node inclusions is one possibility.

Most authors believe that the development of the cysts is actually the result of mechanical obstruction of salivary ducts caused by lymphoid hyperplasia and not due to true de novo cyst formation. The enormous cystic dilatation of the ducts presumably is a consequence of ductal obstruction resulting from hyperplasia of the basal cells of the striated ducts and significant intraglandular lymphofollicular hyperplasia.

BLC occurs almost exclusively in the parotid glands with little or no involvement of the other salivary glands. This may be due to the fact that the parotid gland is the only salivary gland to contain significant lymphoid tissue within it.

The lesions appear on imaging studies as thin-walled cysts in the parotid gland. Sonographic findings, ranging from being purely anechoic to being complex echogenic findings with thick septa and solid components, are nonspecific. However, either CT or MRI demonstrating multiple nonenhancing cysts can suggest the diagnosis. A search for other findings characteristically associated with HIV infection such as lymphoid hyperplasia may be useful in establishing these as HIV-associated lesions.

In the absence of HIV infection, parotid cysts are considered rare. Warthin's tumor or cystic pleomorphic adenoma should be considered in the differential diagnosis if there is a mass associated with the cysts.

The lesions are usually self-limited and surgery is performed for cosmetic reasons or physical discomfort. Some authors advocate enucleation as a safe and effective procedure that provides the patient with complete removal of the cyst and a low recurrence rate.

SUGGESTED READINGS

Finfer MD, Scinella RA, Rothstein SG, et al. Cystic parotid lesions in patients at risk for the acquired immunodeficiency syndrome. *Arch Otolaryngol Head Neck Surg* 1988;114:1290–1294.

Holliday RA, Cohen WA, Schinella RA, et al. Benign lymphoepithelial parotid cysts and hyperplastic cervical adenopathy in AIDS-risk patients: a new CT appearance. *Radiology* 1988;168:439–441.

Mayer M, Haddad J Jr. Human immunodeficiency virus infection presenting with lymphoepithelial cysts in a six-year-old child. *Ann Otol Rhinol Laryngol* 1996;105:242–244.

Schrot RJ, Adelman HM, Linden CN, et al. Cystic parotid gland enlargement in HIV disease. The diffuse infiltrative lymphocytosis syndrome. *JAMA* 1997;9:166–167.

Seddon BM, Padley SP, Gazzard BG. Differential diagnosis of parotid masses in HIV positive men: report of five cases and review. *Int J STD AIDS* 1996;7:224–227.

Som PM, Brandwein MS, Silvers A. Nodal inclusion cysts of the parotid gland and parapharyngeal space: a discussion of lymphoepithelial, AIDS-related parotid, and branchial cysts, cystic Warthin's tumors, and cysts in Sjogren's syndrome. *Laryngoscope* 1995;105:1122–1128.

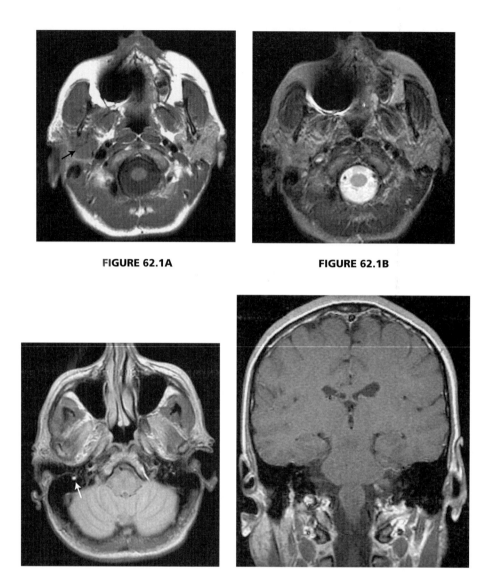

FIGURE 62.1A   FIGURE 62.1B

FIGURE 62.1C   FIGURE 62.1D

CLINICAL HISTORY

Gradual right facial nerve weakness develops in a previously healthy 50-year-old woman.

FINDINGS

Axial T1-weighted MR images through the parotid gland on that side show a parotid mass involving both the superficial and deep lobe of the gland (Fig. 62.1A). On T2-weighted images, it is nearly isointense with the parotid gland (Fig. 62.1B). Axial images above this level following contrast administration show focal enhancement of the mastoid portion of the right facial nerve (Fig. 62.1C). Coronal T1-weighted images postcontrast show a fusiform enlargement and enhancement of the mastoid portion of the facial nerve (Fig. 62.1D).

DIAGNOSIS

Adenoid cystic carcinoma of the parotid gland with perineural extension along the facial nerve into the temporal bone.

DISCUSSION

Adenoid cystic carcinoma is a malignant salivary gland tumor composed of cuboidal cells with a predilection for invading perineural lymphatic spaces. Because of its microscopic appearance, which results in cross sections of tubular cylinders when examined, it was previously referred to as a "cylindroma." The majority of these carcinomas arise from minor salivary glands, but they can also occur in parotid and submandibular glands.

The tumor presents as a superficial parotid mass. Despite its malignant nature, its growth rate is quite slow. Initially, it may be mobile, but with time it becomes indurated and fixed to surrounding tissues. Because of its propensity for perineural spread, facial nerve involvement is not uncommon.

Adenoid cystic carcinoma is a malignant salivary gland tumor that may occur in patients of any age, although it has a peak incidence in the sixth decade. There is a slight female predominance and it is rare in patients younger than 20 years of age. Perineural invasion is a defining feature of this tumor. Thus, the short-term (5-year) survival figures of 70% are misleading. Unlike most other malignancies, recurrences at 10 and 15 years postoperatively are not uncommon with this tumor and the actual cure rate is low.

Perineural extension is a pathway in which the malignant tumor spreads along perineural or endoneural spaces. In this method, tumors can gain access to deep regions that may not be contiguous with the location of the primary tumor. Recognition of this form of extension may alter the form of treatment and prognosis.

The imaging findings of this tumor may be nonspecific and are similar to other parotid neoplasms. Ill-defined margins suggest a more aggressive lesion. Signs of perineural extension should suggest this histology. Fine-needle aspiration cytology has become a valuable tool in the evaluation of these masses. Typical imaging features of perineural spread include smooth thickening of the nerve by an isointense mass, obliteration of adjacent fat, and concentric enlargement of the nerve. Atrophy of muscle groups supplied by the involved cranial nerve is indirect evidence of neural involvement and may be the sole imaging finding.

Parotidectomy is the treatment of choice, with examination of frozen sections for evidence of neural involvement at the time of surgery. The most problematic aspect of the management of adenoid cystic carcinoma is its persistence and tendency to recur locally. Because of radiosensitivity and problems with local control, postoperative radiation is given in many cases.

SUGGESTED READINGS

Huang M, Ma D, Sun K, et al. Factors influencing survival rate in adenoid cystic carcinoma of the salivary glands. *Int J Oral Maxillofac Surg* 1997;26:435–439.

Spiro RH. Distant metastasis in adenoid cystic carcinoma of salivary origin. *Am J Surg* 1997;174:495–498.

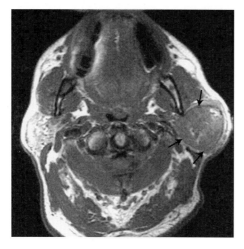

FIGURE 63.1A

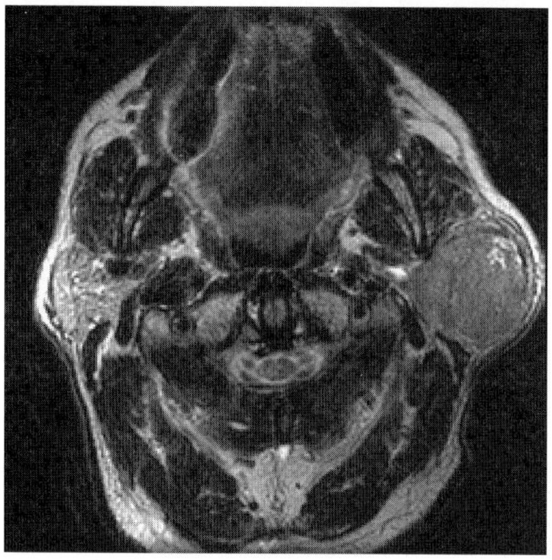

FIGURE 63.1B

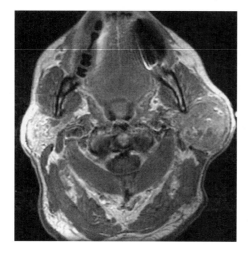

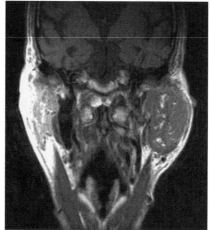

FIGURE 63.1C

FIGURE 63.1D

CLINICAL HISTORY

An elderly woman presents with a painless mass in the left parotid region. The mass has grown slowly over several years.

FINDINGS

The axial T1-weighted image shows a large mass in the left parotid involving both the superficial and deep lobes (Fig. 63.1A). It has a heterogeneous signal intensity both on T1- and T2-weighted images (Fig. 63.1B). It enhances uniformly (Fig. 63.1C). The coronal view shows that there is no invasion of surrounding structures (Fig. 63.1D).

DIAGNOSIS

Oncocytoma of the parotid gland.

DISCUSSION

Oncocytomas, also known as oxyphilic adenoma, oncocytic adenoma, and oxyphilic granular cell adenoma, accounts for less than 1% of all salivary gland tumors and is most commonly found in the parotid gland. The submandibular gland and minor salivary glands are rarely involved but are more likely to harbor aggressive tumors.

Bilateral and multiple tumors occur in up to 7% of cases. Oncocytoma is the second most common cause of multicentric parotid neoplasms following Warthin's tumor. Sometimes, these lesions may obliterate the entire parotid gland. The malignant counterpart of this neoplasm is uncommon, accounting for only 0.005% of all epithelial salivary tumors.

The peak incidence of oncocytomas is between the sixth and seventh decades of life with oncocytic metaplasia of minor salivary glands being not uncommon in the elderly. There is no gender preponderance. Patients with oncocytoma typically present with a painless, slow-growing parotid mass. Bilateral enlargement of the parotid glands is not uncommon and indicates multicentricity. Facial nerve dysfunction and periparotid or cervical lymphadenopathy are both suggestive of malignancy.

The hallmark of this neoplasm is the presence of large cells containing abundant eosinophilic and granular cytoplasm called *oncocytes*. "Onkos" is a Greek word for swelling. Ultrastructural and histochemical studies show that the granular appearance of the cytoplasm is the result of mitochondrial hyperplasia with abnormal rounded shapes, loss of typical architectural features, and bizarre forms, stacking together like erythrocytes in rouleaux.

Oncocytes are not unique to the salivary glands but also occur in other endocrine organs (the thyroid, parathyroid, and pituitary glands) as well as in the kidney. These cells, once thought to arise from a degenerative process, are currently believed to result from redifferentiation of epithelial cells which develop an increased but unbalanced metabolism resulting from an acquired enzymatic defect in the mitochondrial oxidative process. As such, oncocytes are the result of a mitochondriopathy.

Like other benign-appearing parotid neoplasms, the imaging findings of oncocytomas are nonspecific and can be similar to those of a Warthin's tumor or a pleomorphic adenoma. On cross-sectional imaging, they appear as well-circumscribed, homogeneous solid masses that tend to be hypoechoic on ultrasound and hyperdense to the normal parenchyma on CT. On MRI, the signal characteristics are also nonspecific, showing low signal intensity on T1-weighted images and high signal intensity on T2-weighted images.

The diagnosis should be considered when multicentric or bilateral neoplasms are seen in the appropriate clinical setting. The presence of aggressive features such as ill-defined margins, perineural spread, and regional lymphadenopathy suggest malignancy. These lesions are indistinguishable from other more common parotid malignancies.

The most specific imaging study is sialoscintigraphy using technetium-99m pertechnetate. Unlike other salivary cell types, oncocytes are able to concentrate pertechnetate ions, allowing oncocytomas to show intense uptake and retention of radiotracer activity. Thus, sialoscintigraphy helps to differentiate Warthin's tumor and oncocytoma from other benign and malignant salivary gland tumors. It may also localize regional and distant metastasis when a malignant oncocytoma is present.

Some other salivary gland conditions, particularly infection and inflammatory processes, also show increased radionuclide uptake either from hyperemia or retention of the radiotracer in cystic spaces. However, in these circumstances, the uptake is usually diffuse and the clinical history is revealing. Ultimately, fine-needle aspiration is usually performed for tissue diagnosis.

Benign oncocytomas have a good prognosis, and recurrence after complete removal is unusual. Some authors disagree regarding the necessity of resecting asymptomatic parotid lesions in elderly patients because of their very slow growth and the rarity of malignant degeneration.

Malignant oncocytomas require wide resection and radical neck dissection when regional lymph node metastasis is present. The role of adjuvant radiotherapy in the treatment of this rare tumor is unknown. Prognosis is similar to that of other epithelial parotid malignancies.

SUGGESTED READINGS

Ardekian L, Manor R, Peled M, et al. Malignant oncocytoma of the parotid gland: case report and analysis of the literature. *J Oral Maxillofac Surg* 1999;57:325–328.

Davy CL, Dardick I, Hammond E, et al. Relationship of clear cell oncocytoma to mitochondrial-rich (typical) oncocytomas of parotid salivary gland. An ultrastructural study. *Oral Surg Oral Med Oral Pathol* 1994;77:469–479.

Kandiloros D, Segas J, Papadimitriou K, et al. Malignant oncocytoma of the parotid with oncocytic change of the contralateral gland. *Am J Otolaryngol* 1995;16:200–204.

Laforga JB, Aranda FI. Oncocytic carcinoma of parotid gland: fine-needle aspiration and histologic findings. *Diagn Cytopathol* 1994;11:376–379.

Mahnke CG, Jänig U, Werner JA. Metastasizing malignant oncocytoma of the submandibular gland. *J Laryngol Otol* 1998;112:106–109.

Roden DM, Levy FE. Oncocytoma of the parotid gland presenting with nerve paralysis. *Otolaryngol Head Neck Surg* 1994;110:587–590.

San Pedro EC, Lorberboym M, Machac J, et al. Imaging of multiple bilateral parotid gland oncocytomas. *Clin Nucl Med* 1995;20:515–518.

Shintaku M, Honda T. Identification of oncocytic lesions of salivary glands by anti-mitochondrial immunohistochemistry. *Histopathology* 1997;31:408–411.

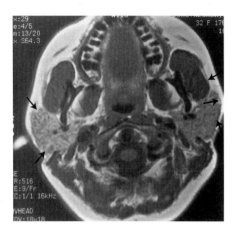

FIGURE 64.1A

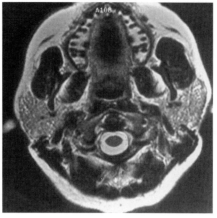

FIGURE 64.1B

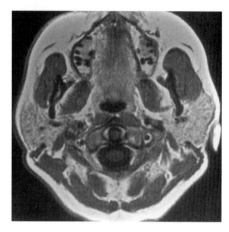

FIGURE 64.1C

CLINICAL HISTORY

A young woman presents with recurrent episodes of bilateral parotid swelling and xerostomia.

FINDINGS

On MRI of the parotid glands, axial T1-weighted image shows bilateral enlargement of the parotid glands and parenchymal heterogeneity with a granular appearance (Fig. 64.1A). The T2-weighted images show that the small micronodules that were hypointense on T1-weighted imaging are high on signal intensity on T2-weighted imaging (Fig. 64.1B). This corresponds to mildly dilated peripheral salivary ducts. On the postcontrast image, they are less apparent (Fig. 64.1C).

DIAGNOSIS

Sjögren's syndrome or autoimmune sialadenitis.

DISCUSSION

Sjögren's syndrome (SS) is a systemic autoimmune disease of the exocrine glands that may occur alone or in association with connective tissue disorders such as rheumatoid arthritis or lupus. The real incidence of the disease is probably underestimated because symptoms may be nonspecific and serologic studies may be negative in the quiescent stages. Autopsy studies show an incidence of 0.4%, placing SS as the second most common autoimmune disease following rheumatoid arthritis.

SS is a chronic inflammatory exocrinopathy affecting primarily the salivary and lacrimal glands. The precise mechanism triggering this autoimmune process is unknown, although Epstein-Barr virus and retroviruses have been postulated as possible candidates. Among the salivary glands, the parotid glands are the most commonly affected. SS is characterized by a diffuse lymphocytic infiltration forming small collections around the intralobular ducts and causing atrophy and replacement of the acinar structures. Concurrently, the ductal epithelium proliferates, obliterating the ductal lumina and producing epithelial islands that may undergo granular metaplasia and hyalinization. The presence of these islands is necessary to establish the histologic diagnosis of benign lymphoepithelial lesion or Godwin's tumor but is not specific for SS. In the later stages, fatty infiltration of the glands becomes a prominent feature. Both the epithelial and lymphoid component of these lesions may undergo malignant transformation, accounting for the increased incidence of lymphoma (44 times higher than in the general population) and epithelial malignancies in patients with SS.

SS is defined by a clinical triad that includes xerostomia, keratoconjunctivitis sicca, and connective tissue disorder. The presence of two or more of these features makes the diagnosis of SS. Most patients present with oral and ocular symptoms including oral dryness and soreness, difficulty swallowing, oral ulcers, multiple recurrent dental caries, and eye dryness and grittiness. Symptoms reflecting involvement of other exocrine glands may also be present such as skin itching, dyspareunia, and nonproductive cough. Xerostomia is a subjective and nonspecific symptom common to other conditions.

The serologic markers of the disease are the SS-A and SS-B antibodies. However, these may only be detected in the active phase of the disease and there are serologically negative forms, particularly in males. The presence of persistent or rapid parotid enlargement along with cervical lymphadenopathy suggests malignant degeneration, most often lymphoma.

Several imaging modalities including sialography, scintigraphy, ultrasound, CT, and MRI may be used and give complementary information. Among these, sialography is considered the "gold standard" in the diagnosis and staging of this disease. Imaging findings depend on the stage of the disease and are more striking in the later stages when cystic degeneration and fatty infiltration predominate. X-ray and MR sialograms may show three different patterns that reflect progressive destructive changes. The earliest stage shows a punctate pattern of numerous peripheral punctate collections of contrast material, less than 1 mm in diameter, uniformly distributed throughout the gland. In the second stage, larger globular collections of contrast material measuring between 1 and 2 mm and resembling a mulberry tree are seen. Finally, the destructive or cavitary pattern shows large, irregular collections of contrast up to 1 cm in diameter, combined with central changes of sialadenitis resulting from ascending infection. In the earlier stages, the uniformity in the size and distribution of the lesions allows differentiation from chronic sialadenitis.

On CT scan, the parotid glands are enlarged and denser than normal (isodense to hyperdense to the masseter muscle). These early findings are nonspecific and are also found in chronic sialadenitis and sialosis. Later, the glands become heterogeneous with an appearance ranging from a micronodular to a honeycombed pattern. A multicystic appearance may be seen similar to that seen with multiple lymphoepithelial cysts, cystic intraparotid lymphadenopathy, multiple abscesses, and multicentric Warthin's tumors. However, in most circumstances, the history and associated clinical findings allow for the differentiation of these conditions. MRI findings are similar to those seen on CT, manifesting as parenchymal heterogeneity, cystic degeneration, and fatty replacement.

Most cases are managed with medical therapy including steroids and, eventually, other immunosuppressors. Parotidectomy is seldom necessary to relieve symptoms of recurrent infection but may be necessary in cases of malignant degeneration.

SUGGESTED READINGS

Izumi M, Eguchi K, Nakamura H, et al. Premature fat deposition in the salivary glands associated with Sjögren syndrome: MR and CT evidence. *AJNR Am J Neuroradiol* 1997;18:951–958.

Izumi M, Eguchi K, Ohki M, et al. MR imaging of the parotid gland in Sjögren's syndrome: a proposal for new diagnostic criteria. *AJR Am J Roentgenol* 1996;166:1483–1487.

Izumi M, Eguchi K, Uetani M, et al. MR features of the lacrimal gland in Sjögren's syndrome. *AJR Am J Roentgenol* 1998;170:1661–1666.

Som PM, Brandwein MS, Silvers A. Nodal inclusion cysts of the parotid gland and parapharyngeal space: a discussion of lymphoepithelial, AIDS-related parotid, and branchial cysts, cystic Warthin's tumors, and cysts in Sjögren's syndrome. *Laryngoscope* 1995;105:1122–1128.

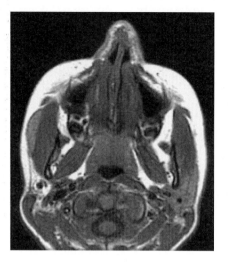

FIGURE 65.1A

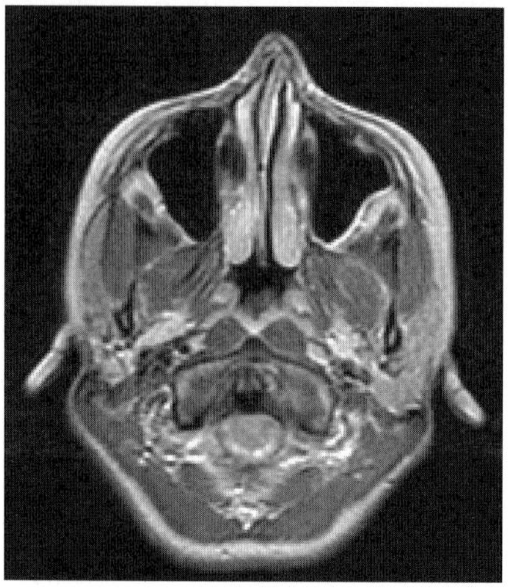

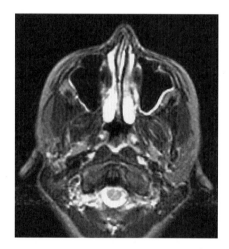

FIGURE 65.1C

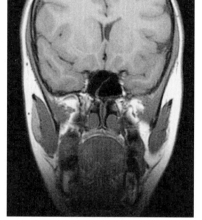

FIGURE 65.1B

FIGURE 65.1D

CLINICAL HISTORY

A 37-year-old man presents with a painless cheek mass. On clinical examination, a nontender, nonmobile, soft mass is palpated in the buccomasseteric region. The facial nerve is intact.

FINDINGS

Axial T1-weighted MRI of the parotid gland shows a soft tissue mass, located laterally to the masseter muscle and caudal to Stenson's duct, following the signal characteristics of the parotid gland parenchyma (Fig. 65.1A). On proton density and T2-weighted images, the lesion follows the signal characteristics of parotid tissue (Fig. 65.1B, C). The ipsilateral parotid gland is absent. There is no evidence of invasion of surrounding structures (Fig. 65.1D).

DIAGNOSIS

Accessory parotid gland.

DISCUSSION

Accessory parotid glands are composed of salivary tissue, which is completely separated from the bulk of the parotid gland proper. It is usually located anterior to the superficial lobe of the parotid gland, lateral to the masseter muscle, and superior to Stenson's duct. It drains into this duct via a variable number of tributary accessory ducts.

Patients usually present with a palpable, painless mass in the cheek, which is frequently felt after some form of facial trauma that calls their attention to that region. On clinical examination, a soft, nontender, and nonmobile mass is palpated within the middle third of a line drawn from the tragus to the inferior border of the nasal ala. The absence of mobility is due to the medial attachment of the accessory parotid tissue to the masseteric fascia. Clinically, the diagnosis is often not readily apparent because the findings mimic any other mass lesion in the masticator or buccal space.

Accessory parotid glands are a frequent finding in the general population. The reported incidence in autopsy studies varies from 20% to 50%. This accessory parotid tissue may be unilateral or bilateral and has a similar incidence in males and females. The size of this accessory parotid tissue is variable but does not generally surpass 3 cm in maximum diameter.

The accessory tissue appears to originate from embryologic remnants of parotid gland tissue that are left over when encapsulation of the gland occurs. Although congenital in origin, this tissue is usually not apparent at birth and grows later in life, eventually presenting in adulthood as a palpable mass.

This salivary tissue is identical to that of the parotid gland of children, containing mixed acini, both serous and mucinous, as opposed to the parotid gland proper in adults, which contains only serous acini. This accessory salivary tissue is susceptible to the same pathologic processes that affect the parotid gland. The most frequent benign neoplasm occurring in the accessory parotid gland is a pleomorphic adenoma. However, the incidence of malignant neoplasms is similar to that of minor salivary glands (approximately 50%) and there is a preponderance of mucoepidermoid carcinoma over adenoid cystic carcinoma, as is seen in children. This again is explained by the histologic composition of the accessory salivary tissue.

Imaging is crucial in the diagnosis of this entity. Ultrasound, CT, and MRI all demonstrate a soft tissue mass lateral to the masseter muscle, anterior and clearly separate from the superficial lobe of the parotid gland, with the same tissue signal characteristics as the parotid gland.

MRI, because of its higher contrast resolution and multiplanar capability, is the method of choice to make the diagnosis in this situation. The normal accessory gland tissue shows the same signal characteristics as the parotid proper on both T1- and T2-weighted images. Accessory parotid gland is frequently an incidental finding on studies performed for unrelated reasons and has no clinical significance other than the potential confusion with pathologic processes. Thus, no therapy is required if there are no pathologic abnormalities in the accessory salivary tissue. Resection may be required for cosmesis. When performing surgery, a preauricular approach is preferred in order to protect the Stenson's duct and the buccal branch of the facial nerve from injury.

SUGGESTED READINGS

Horii A, Honjo Y, Nose M, et al. Accessory parotid gland tumor: a case report. *Auris Nasus Larynx* 1997;24:105–110.

Nemecek JR, Marzek PA, Young VL. Diagnosis and treatment of accessory parotid gland masses. *Ann Plast Surg* 1994;33:75–79.

Tart RP, Kotzur IM, Mancuso AA, et al. CT and MR imaging of the buccal space and buccal space masses. *Radiographics* 1995;15:531–550.

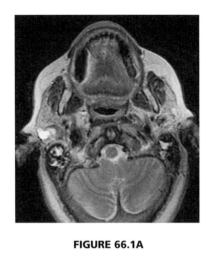

FIGURE 66.1A

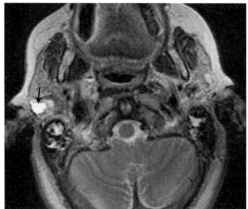

FIGURE 66.1B

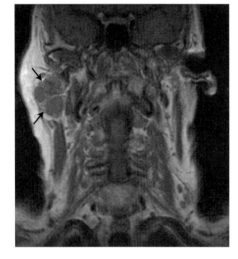

FIGURE 66.1C

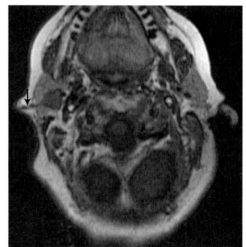

FIGURE 66.1D

CLINICAL HISTORY

An adult male presents with a painless fullness in the face.

FINDINGS

Axial T1-weighted images show a well-circumscribed mass involving both the superficial and deep lobes of the parotid gland (Fig. 66.1A). T2-weighted images show areas of increased signal within the mass, indicating a cystic component (Fig. 66.1B). The coronal views show it to be multiloculated (Fig. 66.1C). Because of the difficulty with directing a needle by clinical palpation, an MR-guided aspiration is performed. The needle is visible as a linear signal void (Fig. 66.1D).

DIAGNOSIS

Warthin's tumor of the parotid gland.

DISCUSSION

Warthin's tumors are the second most common benign tumor of the parotid gland, following pleomorphic adenoma. Warthin's tumors account for 6% to 10% of all parotid gland tumors. The lesions are rare in nonwhite persons and may occur over a wide age range from 2.5 to 92 years, but 82% are found in patients between 40 and 70 years of age with the average being 55 years. Past studies indicate a strong male predominance with a male-to-female ratio of 5:1. However, recent studies suggest that the incidence in women may actually be closer to that in men.

Warthin's tumors are most often located over the angle of the mandible in the tail of the parotid. They usually manifest as a painless mobile mass that may fluctuate in size. Only 10% of patients present with pain and pressure sensations.

Warthin's tumors contain both salivary and lymphoid components with heterotopic salivary gland ductal epithelial elements found in intraparotid or periparotid lymphoid tissues. For this reason, some older textbooks refer to them as cystadenolymphoma or papillary cystadenoma lymphomatosum. Microscopically, these tumors have a double layer of oncocytes that line the papillary projections, which characteristically extend into the cystic spaces.

Warthin's tumors have a greater tendency to undergo cystic changes than any other parotid neoplasms. Clinical fluctuation in size of the tumor is believed to be due to variations in the cystic fluid volume and the degree of lymphoid hyperplasia. With their limited growth potential, most pathologists consider them to be an arising rather than a true neoplasm. Malignant transformation and facial nerve involvement are rare.

Because of the pathogenetic relationship with lymph nodes, Warthin's tumors may also arise in lymph nodes superficial or medial to the parotid gland. Because the parotid is the only salivary gland to contain appreciable lymphoid tissue, this tumor is rare in the submandibular, sublingual, or minor salivary glands. Multiple lesions are not uncommon and they are bilateral in 10% of cases.

On CT, the typical Warthin's tumor is a small, ovoid or lobulated, smoothly marginated mass of homogeneous soft tissue attenuation located most commonly in the posterior aspect of the superficial lobe (the tail) of the parotid gland. Thin-walled cysts are common. The cysts are often of 10 to 20 HU. Focal tumor nodules within the cysts help to distinguish a Warthin's tumor from other cystic lesions such as branchial cleft cysts and lymphangiomas.

On MRI, solid Warthin's tumors are similar to pleomorphic adenomas, demonstrating low T1-weighted and high T2-weighted signal intensities. However, with cystic changes, the cystic fluid usually has sufficiently different signal intensity from the solid component so that the cyst can be identified on some or all of the sequences. Because of this, when small or moderate in size, these tumors tend to be more heterogeneous than pleomorphic adenomas. Occasionally, the cystic nature is not as apparent on MRI as it is on CT. Several other benign or low-grade malignant tumors of the parotid gland could have a similar appearance. In most cases, MRI is not any more accurate than CT in predicting the histologic nature of these parotid tumors.

MRI is not any more accurate than CT in predicting the histologic nature of these parotid tumors. However, a radionuclide scan using technetium 99m-pertechnetate may suggest the diagnosis because technetium is found to accumulate in Warthin's tumor. This is believed to be due to the large number of mitochondria present in the oncocytes within the tumor. Not surprisingly, the only other parotid tumor to show this technetium uptake is oncocytoma.

Simple enucleation is adequate for control of this lesion. However, because of the possibility of multicentricity, most surgeons recommend a superficial or total parotidectomy (depending on the size and location of the lesion) to avoid leaving behind residual disease.

SUGGESTED READINGS

Bruneton JN, Mourou MY. Ultrasound in salivary gland disease. *J Otorhinolaryngol* 1993;55:284–289.

Joe VQ, Westesson PL. Tumors of the parotid gland: MR imaging characteristics of various histologic types. *AJR Am J Roentgenol* 1994;163:433–438.

Minami M, Tanioka H, Oyama K, et al. Warthin tumor of the parotid gland: MR-pathologic correlation. *AJNR Am J Neuroradiol* 1993;14:209–214.

Pinkston JA, Cole P. Incidence rates of salivary gland tumors: results from a population-based study. *Otolaryngol Head Neck Surg* 1999;120:834–840.

Som PM, Brandwein MS, Silvers A. Nodal inclusion cysts of the parotid gland and parapharyngeal space: a discussion of lymphoepithelial, AIDS-related parotid, and branchial cysts, cystic Warthin's tumors, and cysts in Sjogren's syndrome. *Laryngoscope* 1995;105:1122–1128.

Teresi LM, Lufkin RB, Warthan DG, et al. Parotid masses: MR imaging. *Radiology* 1987;163:405–409.

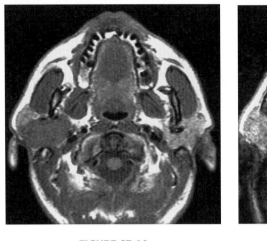

FIGURE 67.1A　　　　**FIGURE 67.1B**

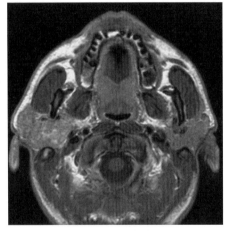

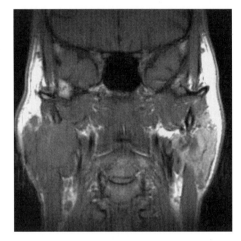

FIGURE 67.1C　　　　**FIGURE 67.1D**

CLINICAL HISTORY

A 35-year-old woman presents with a right-sided facial mass.

FINDINGS

On axial T1-weighted images, a large mass is present in the right parotid gland arising in the superficial lobe and extending for a moderate distance into the deep lobe (Fig. 67.1A). The lesion is heterogeneous on T2-weighted images (Fig. 67.1B). On postcontrast images, the lesion becomes nearly isointense with surrounding tissue (Fig. 67.1C). The coronal image shows the lesion is clear of the skull base superiorly (Fig. 67.1D).

DIAGNOSIS

High-grade mucoepidermoid carcinoma of the right parotid gland.

DISCUSSION

Mucoepidermoid carcinoma is the most common primary malignant tumor of the parotid gland. The tumor typically appears as a focal, well-defined and often movable mass in the superficial portion of the parotid gland. High-grade lesions tend to be more indurated and fixed. Facial nerve weakness is uncommon but, when present, indicates a higher grade lesion.

Mucoepidermoid carcinomas have three predominant cell types: mucous, epidermoid, and intermediate. The behavior of the tumor varies greatly depending on its grade based on its histopathologic features. The low-grade lesions have a preponderance of mucous cells and cystic areas. Although they are unencapsulated or only partially encapsulated, they are generally well circumscribed. Low-grade lesions have limited metastatic potential.

The high-grade lesions have a high proportion of stratified squamous epithelial (epidermoid) cells and may be confused with squamous cell carcinoma. They are aggressive, poorly circumscribed lesions that metastasize to lymph nodes, bone, and lung and have a propensity for perineural spread. The intermediate grade tumors fall between these two extremes.

Imaging findings of mucoepidermoid carcinomas also vary with tumor grade. Low-grade lesions are more "benign" appearing, with a well-delineated, smooth margin. On CT, the appearance is similar to that of a benign mixed tumor. Cystic areas of 10 to 18 HU may be seen. Rarely, focal calcification may be noted. On MRI, these low-grade tumors also have signal intensity that are inseparable from pleomorphic adenomas.

By comparison, the high-grade tumors have indistinct, infiltrative margins. On CT, these lesions usually have few cystic areas and tend to be more homogeneous in appearance than the low-grade tumors. On MRI, the cellular tumors tend to have low to intermediate signal intensity on both T1- and T2-weighted images.

Several authors have attempted to histopathologically distinguish various parotid lesions based on their MR signal characteristics, but without success. Therefore, aspiration cytology is required for most parotid lesions. Whenever malignancy is a possibility, the course of the facial nerve should be included in the study to avoid missing perineural spread of tumor.

Surgery with wide local excision is the treatment of choice for mucoepidermoid carcinoma, employing wide local excision. Neck dissections are generally not performed for low or intermediate grade tumors unless cervical metastases are present. For high-grade tumors, some authors advocate elective neck dissection followed by postoperative radiotherapy.

In most studies, the 5-year survival rate for low-grade lesions is more than 90% and decreases to 50% to 70% for high-grade tumors. The prognosis is dismal for those who present with facial nerve paralysis, with only a 9% to 14% survival rate at 5 years.

SUGGESTED READINGS

Curtin HD. Assessment of salivary gland pathology. *Otolaryngol Clin North Am* 1988;21:547–573.

Goode RK, Auclair PL, Ellis GL. Mucoepidermoid carcinoma of the major salivary glands: clinical and histopathologic analysis of 234 cases with evaluation of grading criteria. *Cancer* 1998;82:1217–1224.

Plambeck K, Friedrich RD, Schmetzle R. Mucoepidermoid carcinoma of the salivary gland origin: classification, clinico-pathological correlation, treatment results and long term follow-up in 55 patients. *J Craniomaxillofac Surg* 1996;24:133–139.

Swartz JD, Rothman MI, Marlowe FI. MR imaging of parotid mass lesions: attempts at histopathologic differentiation. *J Comput Assist Tomogr* 1989;13:789–796.

Teresi LM, Lufkin RB, Wortham DG, et al. Parotid masses: MR imaging. *Radiology* 1987;163:405–409.

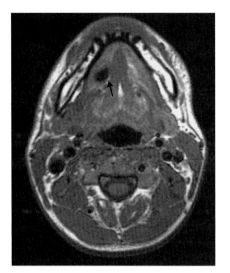

FIGURE 68.1A

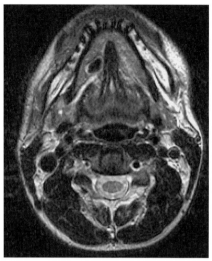

FIGURE 68.1B

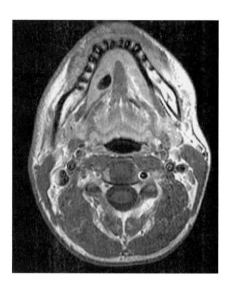

FIGURE 68.1C

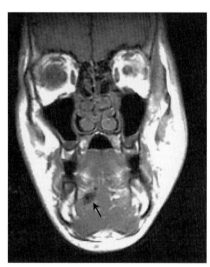

FIGURE 68.1D

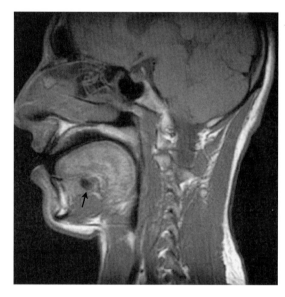

FIGURE 68.1E

CLINICAL HISTORY

The patient presents with swelling in the left floor of mouth region that is exacerbated with eating.

FINDINGS

Axial T1-weighted MR scan shows a focal area of low signal intensity in the region of the left floor of mouth along Warton's duct of the submandibular gland (Fig. 68.1A). On T2-weighted image, this area remains low signal intensity (Fig. 68.1B). On the postcontrast image, there is no evidence of enhancement (Fig. 68.1C). The coronal and sagittal T1-weighted image confirms the position of the mass along the course of Warton's duct (Fig. 68.1D, E).

DIAGNOSIS

Sialolithiasis of the left submandibular gland.

DISCUSSION

Patients with sialolithiasis often present with pain and swelling of the gland, associated with eating. Although when a patient presents with these obstructing symptoms, the other possibility to consider is floor of mouth squamous cell carcinoma. Small stones may also be entirely asymptomatic.

More than 80% of salivary gland stones are found in the submandibular gland. Ten to fifteen percent occur in the parotid gland and the remainder occur in the sublingual glands. Most are solitary with less than 25% being multiple. The three common locations of submandibular sialolithiasis are the ductal opening into the mouth (30%), the posterior edge of the myohyoid muscle (35%), and the midportion of the duct (25%). A stone within the gland itself or the hilum is rare.

The higher incidence of submandibular stones is believed to be due to several factors:

1. More alkaline pH of submandibular saliva, which tends to precipitate salts.
2. Thicker more mucous-like submandibular saliva.
3. Higher concentration in submandibular saliva of hydroxyapatite and phosphatase.
4. Narrower Wharton duct orifice compared with the main lumen.
5. Slight uphill direction of salivary flow in Wharton's duct in the upright position.

Approximately 80% of salivary gland stones are radiopaque. The radiologic study should start with either plain films (anteroposterior, lateral, submental view) or limited CT. Sialographic findings of sialolithiasis are contrast-filling defect and ductal dilatation, if the duct is obstructed. Because CT is much more sensitive in detecting a tiny focus of calcium compared with plain radiographs, thin section CT scan is increasingly being used for patients with suspected salivary gland stones. CT usually reveals high-density stones with or without proximal ductal dilatation. A mimic of submandibular gland stones on CT is unilateral calcification of the stylohyoid ligament.

Because of the lower sensitivity of MR compared with x-ray for the detection of calcification, MR is less well suited for the primary evaluation of patients with this disease. Larger stones may be seen on MR as discrete areas of signal void. However, some centers are performing MR sialography, using heavily T2-weighted fast spin echo (FSE) sequences to allow for detection of ductile declaration and filling defects within the duct in a noninvasive fashion and with good correlation with conventional sialography. Ultrasound has been receiving growing attention as a technique for the evaluation of sialolithiasis. Endoscopy of the salivary ducts has also been reported.

Management depends on the location and the size of stones. A small stone may spontaneously pass with the flow of saliva. Some stones may be removed with a endoluminal approach. Larger ones close to the duct orifice can often be removed by intraoral approach. Stones within the central Warton duct may need total submandibulectomy. An interesting new approach that has been described is to use shock wave lithotripsy to destroy the stones.

SUGGESTED READINGS

Fischbach R, Kugel H, Ernst S, et al. MR sialography: initial experience using a T2-weighted fast SE sequence. *J Comput Assist Tomogr* 1997;21:826–830.

Nahlieli O, Baruchin AM. Sialoendoscopy: three years' experience as a diagnostic and treatment modality. *J Oral Maxillofac Surg* 1997;55:912–918;discussion, 919–920.

Ottaviani F, Capaccio P, Rivolta R, et al. Salivary gland stones: US evaluation in shock wave lithotripsy. *Radiology* 1997;204:437–441.

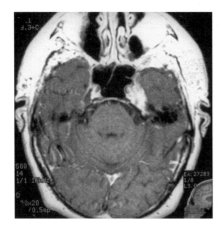

FIGURE 69.1

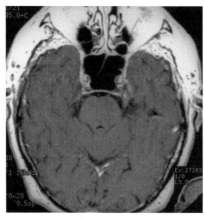

FIGURE 69.2

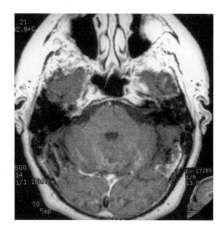

FIGURE 69.3

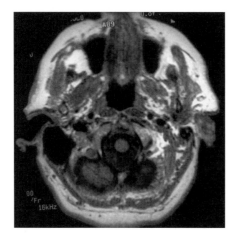

FIGURE 69.4

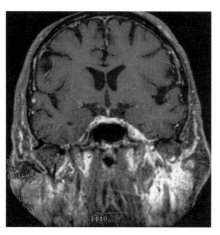

FIGURE 69.5

CLINICAL HISTORY

A 78-year-old man has an 8-month history of left trigeminal and facial nerve symptoms. No visible or palpable mass is seen by otolaryngologic examination.

FINDINGS

Postcontrast T1-weighted image shows an enhancing mass in the left cavernous sinus extending to the prepontine segment of the trigeminal nerve (Fig. 69.1). In addition, subtle contrast enhancement of the greater petrosal nerve is evident on the left (Figs. 69.2, 69.3). No primary head and neck tumor was detected at this time. Six months later, follow-up MRI revealed an ill-defined hypointense mass in the left parotid gland with extension to the masticator space. Contrast-enhanced fat-suppressed coronal image clearly shows extension of the skull base tumor to the trigeminal nerve through the foramen ovale (Fig. 69.4). Note the asymmetric atrophy of the left masticator muscles, indicating left trigeminal nerve involvement (Fig. 69.5).

DIAGNOSIS

Adenoid cystic carcinoma of the parotid gland with perineural extension.

DISCUSSION

This case illustrates an imaging presentation of perineural extension of neoplasm before identifying a primary site. Adenoid cystic carcinoma of the parotid gland may extend along the facial nerve and greater petrosal nerve. The greater petrosal nerve connects with the lateral posterior aspect of the third branch of the trigeminal nerve at the skull base. From the trigeminal nerve, the tumor spreads to the cavernous sinus as well as prepontine segment of the trigeminal nerve.

Perineural tumor spread is a manifestation of direct spread of a primary tumor along perineural and endoneural tissue planes, principally along a "path of least resistance." Recognition of this type of tumor spread may alter the form of treatment and prognosis. Perineural tumor spread can be seen in adenoid cystic carcinoma as well as other tumors of the extracranial head and neck, including squamous cell carcinoma, lymphoma, other minor salivary tumors, melanoma, chondrosarcomas, malignant schwannomas, and other sarcomas. Perineural spread of tumor should be included in the differential diagnosis of a cavernous sinus mass lesion.

Tumors may spread centrally or peripherally along a cranial nerve and may involve their cisternal segments and spread to the brainstem. Typical MR features of perineural spread include smooth thickening of the nerve by an isointense mass, obliteration of adjacent fat, and concentric enlargement of basal foramina associated with a distant mass that may or may not be contiguous. Atrophy of muscle groups supplied by the involved cranial nerve is indirect evidence of neural involvement but may be the only finding. Gadolinium-enhanced MRI with or without fat suppression is superior to CT in the demonstration of perineural tumor in the cavernous sinus and preganglionic segment of the trigeminal nerve. Because perineural tumor represents direct extension of tumor, recognition of this entity is crucial for complete surgical resection or radiotherapy planning. Negative imaging studies should not deter surgeons from nerve sheath biopsy in patients with appropriate history and symptoms.

SUGGESTED READINGS

Batsakis JG. Nerves and neurotropic carcinomas. *Ann Otol Rhinol Laryngol* 1985;94:426–427.

Curtin HD, Williams R, Johnson J. CT of perineural tumor extension: pterygopalatine fossa. *Am J Neuroradiol* 1984;5:731–737.

Ginsberg LE. Imaging of perineural tumor spread in head and neck cancer. *Semin Ultrasound CT MR* 1999;20:175–186.

Harnsberger HR, Dillon WP. Major motor atrophic patterns in the face and neck: CT evaluation. *Radiology* 1985;155:665–670.

Laine FJ, Braun IF, Jensen ME, et al. Perineural tumor extension through the foramen ovale: evaluation with MR imaging. *Radiology* 1990;174:65–71.

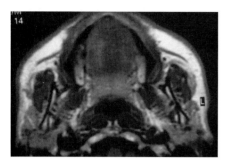

FIGURE 70.1A

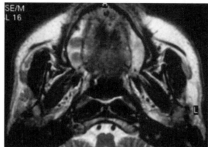

FIGURE 70.1B

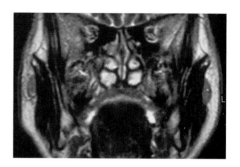

FIGURE 70.1C

CLINICAL HISTORY

A 58-year-old man has a long history of bilateral, nontender buccomasseteric masses. On clinical examination, rounded, nonmobile masses are palpated over the masseter muscles.

FINDINGS

Axial T1- and T2-weighted and coronal T2-weighted images through the parotid glands show bilateral small masses located laterally to the masseter muscles and cephalad to Stenson's duct. The masses are separate from the bulk of the parotid gland and follow the signal characteristics of the parotid gland parenchyma in all pulse sequences (Fig. 70.1A–C).

DIAGNOSIS

Bilateral accessory parotid glands.

DISCUSSION

Accessory parotid gland and facial process of the parotid gland are the most frequent causes of unilateral buccomasseteric masses. The buccomasseteric region includes the masseter and buccinator muscles, the buccal space, and the inferior portion of the mandibular body. In most individuals, the superficial lobe of the parotids overlie the posterior third of the masseter muscle. The Stenson's duct, after exiting the gland parenchyma, courses lateral to the masseter and enters the buccal fat pad before piercing the buccinator muscle at the level of the second maxillary molar. However, in some individuals, parotid gland tissue extends anteriorly as far as the buccinator muscle and this normal variant is referred to as *facial process of the parotid gland.* Accessory parotid gland implies the presence of a bulk of parotid tissue separate from the parotid gland proper, usually located anteriorly to the superficial lobe of the parotid gland and above the level of Stenson's duct.

This accessory salivary tissue is thought to result from remnants of parotid tissue that are left over during embryologic encapsulation of the parotid gland. Although considered a congenital entity, accessory parotid glands do not present during childhood. During adulthood, as salivary tissue grows, they become evident. The incidence of accessory parotid glands ranges from 20% to 50% according to different series and may be unilateral or bilateral. Because it carries no pathologic consequences, this situation is considered by most to be a normal variant, although accessory parotid tissue may be the site for any of the pathologic processes arising from salivary gland tissue. Like for minor salivary glands, tumors arising from accessory parotids have a 50% chance of being malignant.

Imaging features on both CT and MRI are almost pathognomonic, showing a well-defined mass in the buccomasseteric region that follows the same density and intensity of eutopic parotid tissue and shares the same tissue architecture. In questionable cases, sialography may be valuable in that it demonstrates small accessory parotid ducts draining into Stenson's duct.

Differential diagnosis of unilateral masses in the bucco-masseteric region includes Stenson's duct dilation or sialocele, buccal space lymphadenopathy and abscess, pedunculated tumors arising from the superficial lobe of the parotid gland, and several benign tumors such as hemangioma, lymphangioma, lipoma, and rhabdomyoma, and their malignant counterparts.

No therapy is required, but surgical resection may be performed for cosmesis.

SUGGESTED READINGS

Arata H, Yuichiro H, Michihiro N, et al. Accessory parotid gland tumor: a case report. *Aurus Nasis Larynx* 1997;24:105–110.

Batsakis JG. Pathology consultation: accessory parotid gland. *Ann Otol Rhinol Laryngol* 1998;97:434–435.

Frommer J. The human accessory parotid gland: its incidence, nature and significance. *Oral Surg* 41997;3:671–676.

Nemecek JR, Marzek PA, Young VL. Diagnosis and treatment of accessory parotid gland masses. *Ann Plast Surg* 1994;33:75–80.

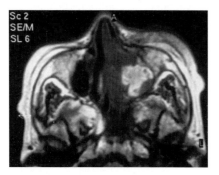

FIGURE 71.1A   **FIGURE 71.1B**

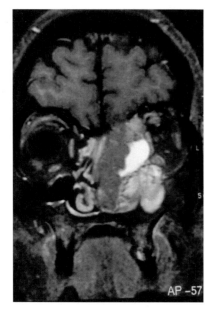

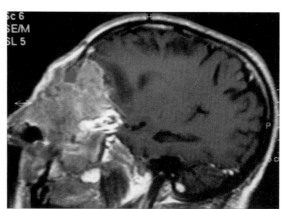

FIGURE 71.1C   **FIGURE 71.2**

CLINICAL HISTORY

The patient is a 72-year-old woman with a longstanding history of unilateral nasal obstruction and recent onset of epistaxis and left-sided proptosis.

FINDINGS

There is a large heterogeneous mass in the left nasoethmoidal region. The lesion fills the left nasal fossa and extends posteriorly into the left choana and laterally into the extraconal compartment of the left orbit pushing the medial rectus and optic nerve and leading to proptosis. Superiorly, the mass abuts and destroys the cribriform plate, slightly bulging into the anterior cranial fossa. There is no abnormal dural enhancement and no evidence of invasion of the brain parenchyma. The mass is heterogeneous in signal intensity, showing speckled areas of hemorrhage and heterogeneous contrast enhancement. There are extensive postobstructive changes with opacification of the ipsilateral maxillary antrum, sphenoid, and frontal sinuses by hyperintense material on both T1- and T2-weighted images, suggesting fluid with high protein content (Fig. 71.1A, axial T1-weighted image; 71.1B, axial T2-weighted image; 71.1C, coronal fat-suppressed postcontrast T1-weighted image).

Figure 71.2 shows sagittal postcontrast T1-weighted image of another patient with a nasofrontoethmoidal lesion with bilateral orbital and intracranial invasion.

DIAGNOSIS

Squamous cell carcinoma of the nasoethmoidal region.

DISCUSSION

Sinonasal carcinomas are rare tumors of the head and neck. Most are of epithelial origin (50%), followed in decreasing order of frequency by adenocarcinomas, lymphomas, malignancies arising from minor salivary glands, melanomas, and sarcomas. The maxillary sinus is most commonly involved (70% of cases) followed by the nasal cavity (20%), ethmoid complex (10%), and the sphenoid and frontal sinuses (<1%). There is a peak incidence in the sixth decade and a slight male predilection.

Several predisposing factors have been identified in the pathogenesis of sinonasal neoplasms. Occupational exposure to several irritants, and previous exposure to radiation and thorotrast have all been implicated. Inverting papilloma is also associated with an incidence of 15% to 20% of synchronous or metachronous squamous cell carcinoma of the sinonasal tract. Less established predisposing factors include chronic sinusitis, sinonasal polyposis, and chronic nasoantral fistulas.

Because the site of origin and pattern of tumor spread have crucial prognostic and therapeutic implications, several systems have been developed to classify squamous cell carcinoma of the paranasal sinuses. Ohngren subdivided the sinonasal region using an imaginary line joining the medial canthus with the angle of the mandible into a superior portion that he called the suprastructure and an inferior portion or infrastructure. This division separates tumors that are either not resectable or require wide craniofacial resections from tumors that are amenable to less radical surgery and that also have a much better prognosis.

Squamous cell carcinoma of the nasoethmoid region has a poor prognosis, with most patients presenting late in the course of the disease with orbital or intracranial invasion. Symptoms and signs are often confused with inflammatory and infectious processes and, not uncommonly, chronic rhinosinusitis is diagnosed. Unilateral nasal stuffiness and epistaxis in an adult patient should be viewed with suspicion requiring a thorough ear, nose, and throat evaluation and imaging studies.

Cross-sectional imaging is the only reliable method for evaluation of tumor extent and is mandatory for treatment planning. The radiologist's role is to provide accurate tumor mapping and detect critical areas of involvement that may alter the treatment modality or surgical approach. In the case of tumors arising in the nasal vault or ethmoid complex, crucial regions include the orbits and intracranial extension. Although CT may be slightly better in detecting bony erosion of the lamina papyracea and cribriform plate, MRI is definitely superior to evaluate the extension of the soft tissue component, allowing separation between tumor and postobstructive changes. Also, intraorbital and intracranial extent must be evaluated on postgadolinium MR images in several planes. The imaging features are nonspecific, usually demonstrating a destructive, invasive mass that is hypointense to isointense on T1-weighted images, hyperintense on T2-weighted images (less so than postobstructive inflammatory changes), and enhance on postcontrast images.

Fat-suppressed, T1-weighted, gadolinium-enhanced images are the sequence of choice to evaluate intraorbital extent separating neoplastic tissue from the intraconal and extraconal orbital fat. Meningeal invasion is not uncommon and manifests as intense dural enhancement.

Differential diagnosis includes other malignant neoplasms such as adenocarcinoma, lymphoma, minor salivary gland neoplasms, esthesioneuroblastoma, and sarcomas. These cannot be distinguished from squamous cell carcinoma on imaging basis. Melanoma of the sinonasal region is another consideration. MRI may suggest this diagnosis when the typical signal characteristics of melanin are found (hyperintensity on T1-weighted images).

Aggressive infections including fungal sinusitis, bacterial osteomyelitis, and rhinoscleroma can also be mistaken for neoplasms when associated with bony destructive changes. Nodal metastases are rare because the paranasal sinuses have a poor lymphatic network. However, these tumors are locally aggressive and curative treatment is difficult to achieve.

SUGGESTED READINGS

Alvarez I, Suarez C, Rodrigo JP, et al. Prognostic factors in paranasal sinus cancer. *Am J Otolaryngol* 1995;16:109–114.

Carinci F, Curioni C, Padula E, et al. Cancer of the nasal cavity and paranasal sinuses: a new staging system. *Int J Maxillofac Surg* 1996;25:34–39.

Jacobsen MH, Larsen SK, Kirkegaard J, et al. Cancer of the nasal cavity and paranasal sinuses: prognosis and outcome of treatment. *Acta Oncol* 1997;36:28–31.

Lesperance MM, Esclamado RM. Squamous cell carcinoma arising in inverted papilloma. *Laryngoscope* 1995;105:178–183.

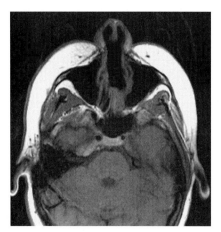

FIGURE 72.1A

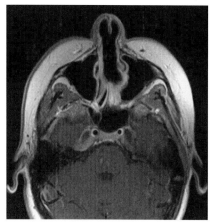

FIGURE 72.1B

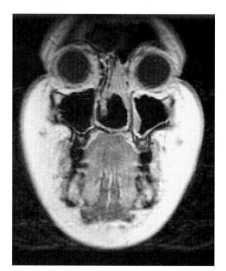

FIGURE 72.1C

CLINICAL HISTORY

A 44-year-old man presents with nasal obstruction and chronic purulent rhinorrhea. The patient denies cocaine use.

FINDINGS

The axial T1-weighted MR scan shows mucosal thickening of the maxillary sinuses bilaterally and a prominent septal perforation (Fig. 72.1A). The axial T2-weighted and coronal images confirm these findings (Fig. 72.1B, C).

DIAGNOSIS

Nasal lymphoma.

DISCUSSION

In 1939, Wegener described a "rhinogenic granulomatosis" in patients with necrotizing granulomatous vasculitis of the upper and lower respiratory tract and kidneys. The lungs are involved in nearly all cases.

After exclusion of the Wegener's granulomatosis patients, the remaining group of patients with idiopathic aggressive destructive nasal lesions were known in the 1950s and 1960s as having "lethal midline granuloma." This was a particularly poor choice of terms because it became clear that, although the disease was almost always midline, it was not always lethal or granulomatous.

In the 1970s and 1980s, patients with this disorder were subclassified into the following three groups based on varia-

tions in histology and clinical behavior:

1. Idiopathic midline destructive disease characterized by localized destructive lesion of the nasal cavity with non-specific inflammation and necrosis.
2. Polymorphic reticulosis or lymphomatoid granulomatosis with a pseudolymphomatous tissue reaction.
3. Extranodal lymphoma, usually non-Hodgkin's type

Finally, in the 1990s, advances in immunocytochemical phenotyping allowed a great simplification in the understanding of this disease. The vast majority of patients from the previous groups are currently known to have lymphoma of the nasal tract. The use of the previous nomenclature to describe these sinonasal lymphomas should be discontinued. The following terms should no longer be used:

Lethal midline granuloma
Idiopathic midline destructive disease
Polymorphic reticulosis
Lymphomatoid granulomatosis
Pseudolymphoma
Stewart's granuloma

Nasal lymphoma is one of the more uncommon forms of extranodal lymphoma in Western populations, representing less than 0.5% of the group. In contrast, in Asia, sinonasal lymphoma is the second most common type of extranodal lymphoma, exceeded only by those in the gastrointestinal system. The median age of patients at diagnosis is 50 years.

Nasal obstruction or purulent nasal discharge are frequent presenting symptoms. Epistaxis and facial swelling are also sometimes seen. Eventually, septal perforation, sinonasal-oral fistulas, and even "autorhinectomy" may develop.

In early cases, CT or MR studies show nonspecific sinonasal findings of mucosal thickening suggesting chronic sinonasal inflammation. Eventually, destructive lesions appear, with septal perforation and occasionally sinonasal oral fistulas. The destructive nasal imaging findings may be identical to those seen in Wegener's granulomatosis. With advanced disease, complete nasal destruction (autorhinectomy) may occur in either this disease or in Wegener's patients.

Radiation therapy is the treatment of choice, although some authors use chemotherapy alone or in combination with radiation therapy.

SUGGESTED READINGS

Borisch B, Hennig I, Laeng RH, et al. Association of the subtype 2 of the Epstein-Barr virus with T-cell non-Hodgkin's lymphoma of the midline granuloma type. *Blood* 1993;82:858–864.

Ramsay AD, Rooney N. Lymphomas of the head and neck. 1: Nasofacial T-cell lymphoma. *Eur J Cancer B Oral Oncol* 1993;29B:99–102.

Chen HH, Fong L, Su IJ, et al. Experience of radiotherapy in lethal midline granuloma with special emphasis on centrofacial T-cell lymphoma: a retrospective analysis covering a 34-year period. *Radiother Oncol* 1996;38:1–6.

Dictor M, Cervin A, Kalm O, et al. Sinonasal T-cell lymphoma in the differential diagnosis of lethal midline granuloma using in situ hybridization for Epstein-Barr virus RNA. *Mod Pathol* 1996;9:7–14.

Hartig G, Montone K, Wasik M, et al. Nasal T-cell lymphoma and the lethal midline granuloma syndrome. *Otolaryngol Head Neck Surg* 1996;114:653–656.

Sevinsky LD, Woscoff A, Jaimovich L, et al. Nasal cocaine abuse mimicking midline granuloma. *J Am Acad Dermatol* 1995;32(2 Pt 1):286–287.

CASE 73

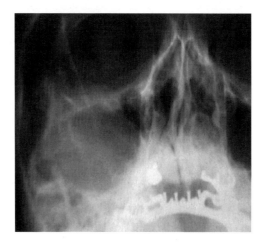

FIGURE 73.1A

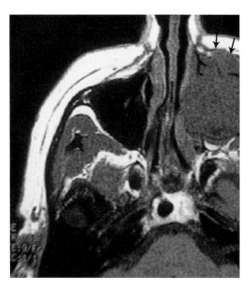

FIGURE 73.1B

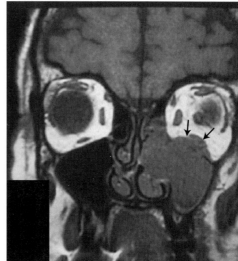

FIGURE 73.1C

CLINICAL HISTORY

A 50-year-old man with a longstanding history of chronic sinusitis presents with left facial swelling.

FINDINGS

Plain film Water's view of the sinus shows a soft tissue mass in the floor of the maxillary sinus with associated bone destruction of the inferolateral wall (Fig. 73.1A). Axial MR section of a similar patient shows the mass with bony destruction and extension into the anterior soft tissues of the face (Fig. 73.1B). The coronal T1-weighted image shows invasion into the orbit by the mass (Fig. 73.1C).

DIAGNOSIS

Squamous carcinoma of the maxillary sinus.

168

DISCUSSION

Sinonasal carcinomas are detected late in the course of the disease because symptoms (nasal stuffiness, sinonasal fullness, and nasal quality of voice) are nonspecific and frequently mimic common benign diseases such as chronic sinusitis or sinonasal polyposis. Also, these inflammatory and infectious processes usually arise as a result of an underlying neoplasm overshadowing and delaying the diagnosis. Unilateral nasal obstruction and epistaxis in an adult patient strongly suggests the diagnosis. Most cases, however, present with symptoms reflecting invasion of adjacent structures such as facial swelling, diplopia, orbital pain, proptosis, decreasing vision, and headache. Spread of tumor to the masticator space and nasolacrimal duct is not rare and may present with trismus and epiphora, respectively. On physical examination, the most common finding is a nasal mass. Visual field defects, decreased visual acuity, and cranial nerve deficits (usually cranial nerve V) can occur. Sinonasal endoscopy is not reliable for evaluation of tumor extent.

Sinonasal carcinomas are rare, comprising only 3% of all head and neck tumors. Among these, approximately 50% are of epithelial origin. The maxillary antrum is most commonly involved (80% of cases), followed in decreasing order of frequency by the nasal cavity (20%), ethmoid complex (10%), and sphenoid and frontal sinuses (<1%). There is a male predisposition with a male-to-female ratio of 2:1 and a peak incidence in the sixth decade. Ninety percent of cases are seen in patients older than 40 years. In the pediatric population, most destructive sinonasal masses are either rhabdomyosarcomas or eosinophilic granulomas.

Several predisposing factors have been implicated in the pathogenesis of sinonasal neoplasms. Occupational exposure to irritants such as nickel, chromium, wood furniture, mustard gas, and radium are associated with an increased incidence of carcinomas, mostly squamous cell and adenocarcinoma. An increased incidence of sinonasal carcinoma and sarcoma is also seen in patients previously exposed to radiation and thorotrast. Fifteen to twenty-five percent of patients with inverting papilloma have synchronous or metachronous squamous cell carcinoma. Other less established causative factors include chronic sinusitis, sinonasal polyposis, and chronic nasoantral fistulas. The association with airborne agents explains the increased incidence of sinonasal carcinomas in the nasal cavity and maxillary antra, the first barrier to inhaled irritants.

Because the site of origin and pattern of tumor spread have prognostic and therapeutic impact, several systems have been used to classify squamous cell carcinoma of the paranasal sinuses, most regarding antral tumors, the most prevalent location. In 1933, Ohngren subdivided the maxillary antrum into a suprastructure and infrastructure using an imaginary line joining the medial canthus with the angle of the mandible. Neoplasms located posterosuperior to this line are either unresectable or require wide craniofacial re-

sections, usually total maxillectomy with orbital exenteration, and have a grave prognosis (10% 5-year survival rate). Tumors located anteroinferior to this line can be managed with partial or total maxillectomy and have a better prognosis (58% 5-year survival rate).

The tumor, node, metastases (TNM) classification is based in Ohngren's line and classifies maxillary neoplasms as follows:

T1—Tumor limited to the antral mucosa.
T2—Bony erosion with no extension beyond the bone.
T3—Extension into the orbit, ethmoidal region, or premaxillary soft tissues.
T4—Extension into the nasopharynx, sphenoid sinus, cribriform plate, or pterygopalatine fossa.

Because the lymphatic drainage of the paranasal sinuses is poor, nodal metastasis is uncommon (15%) and usually indicates spread of tumor beyond the boundaries of the maxillary sinus, most commonly into the alveolar sulcus, pterygopalatine fossa, or premaxillary soft tissues. The primary lymphatic drainage of the paranasal sinuses is to the retropharyngeal lymph nodes. However, because this lymphatic pathway is often obliterated as a result of repeated childhood infections, the secondary lymph nodes (high internal jugular chain and submandibular nodes) are the most commonly involved.

Cross-sectional imaging is the only reliable method to evaluate tumor extent, allowing more precise treatment planning. The radiologist's role is to provide accurate tumor mapping and detect critical areas of involvement, which may alter either the treatment modality or the surgical approach. In the case of a maxillary tumor, these critical areas include the orbits, pterygopalatine fossa, anterior and middle cranial fossa, maxillary alveolar ridge, and palate.

MRI and CT are complementary and together can provide adequate mapping of both soft tissue and bony involvement. Antral neoplasms present as poorly enhancing soft tissue masses, usually extending beyond the boundaries of the sinus of origin. On CT, it may be difficult to differentiate neoplasm from postobstructive inflammatory changes on the basis of differential attenuation values. T2-weighted MRI is used to separate the intermediate signal intensity of neoplasm from the bright signal intensity of inflammatory material. Squamous cell carcinoma tends to be fairly homogeneous, although large tumors may contain areas of necrosis or hemorrhage. Small tumors often escape both clinical and radiologic detection. The only imaging criteria that suggest malignancy are the presence of aggressive bony changes or enlarged lymph nodes, both signaling advanced disease. Imaging follow-up is mandatory for detection of recurrence or residual tumor and a baseline, posttherapy scan should be obtained for future comparison.

Treatment of sinonasal carcinoma depends on the stage of the disease. For most T3 and T4 tumors, the treatment options are radiation therapy or wide craniofacial resections. Although there is more morbidity associated with surgery, especially in terms of facial disfigurement, most studies have shown a better survival rate in patients who underwent surgery. T1 and T2 tumors are managed surgically with total or partial maxillectomy.

SUGGESTED READINGS

Alvarez I, Suárez C, Rodrigo JP, et al. Prognostic factors in paranasal sinus cancer. *Am J Otolaryngol* 1995;16:109–114.

Carinci F, Curioni C, Padula E, et al. Cancer of the nasal cavity and paranasal sinuses: a new staging system. *Int J Oral Maxillofac Surg* 1996;25:34–39.

Harbo G, Grau C, Bundgaard T, et al. Cancer of the nasal cavity and paranasal sinuses. A clinico-pathological study of 277 patients. *Acta Oncol* 1997;36:45–50.

Houston GD. Sinonasal undifferentiated carcinoma: report of two cases and review of the literature. *Oral Surg Oral Med Oral Pathol Oral Radiol Endod* 1998;85:185–188.

Jakobsen MH, Larsen SK, Kirkegaard J, et al. Cancer of the nasal cavity and paranasal sinuses. Prognosis and outcome of treatment. *Acta Oncol* 1997;36:27–31.

Lesperance MM, Esclamado RM. Squamous cell carcinoma arising in inverted papilloma. *Laryngoscope* 1995;105:178–183.

Parsons JT, Kimsey FC, Mendenhall WM, et al. Radiation therapy for sinus malignancies. *Otolaryngol Clin North Am* 1995;28:1259–1268.

Som PM, Silvers AR, Catalano PJ, et al. Adenosquamous carcinoma of the facial bones, skull base, and calvaria: CT and MR manifestations. *AJNR Am J Neuroradiol* 1997;18:173–175.

Wennerberg J. Pre versus post-operative radiotherapy of resectable squamous cell carcinoma of the head and neck. *Acta Otolaryngol* 1995;115:465–474.

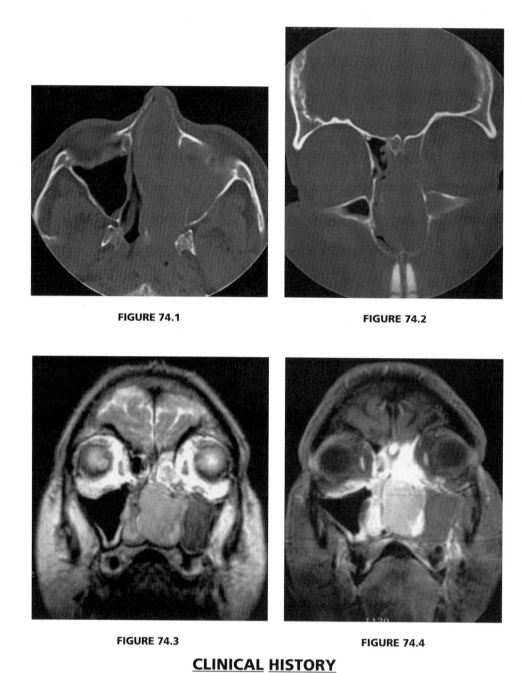

FIGURE 74.1

FIGURE 74.2

FIGURE 74.3

FIGURE 74.4

CLINICAL HISTORY

An 82-year-old woman presents with a 6- to 12-month history of nasal obstruction.

FINDINGS

Maxillofacial CT shows a large expansile mass occupying the left nasal cavity associated with rightward bowing of the nasal septum (Fig. 74.1). The left maxillary, ethmoid, and sphenoid sinuses are opacified with soft tissue attenuation. The medial inferior orbital wall (lamina papyracea) is eroded by the left nasal mass (Fig. 74.2). T2-weighted MR image shows the left nasal mass being lower in signal compared with the inflamed sinonasal mucosa (Fig. 74.3). Postcontrast image reveals enhancing tumor, clearly differentiating a tumor from obstructed paranasal sinuses (Fig. 74.4).

DIAGNOSIS

Nasal lymphoma.

DISCUSSION

Malignant neoplasms of the paranasal sinuses and nasal cavity are uncommon lesions, accounting for less than 0.8% of all malignancies and approximately 3% of cancers involving the upper aerodigestive tract. Sinonasal lymphoma (non-Hodgkin's lymphoma) is a rare disease and most cases occur in the nasal cavity or maxillary sinus, and less often in the ethmoid sinus. Associated cervical lymphadenopathy is relatively uncommon, but if it occurs, it usually represents poor prognosis. Retropharyngeal, submandibular, and jugular lymph nodes may be involved in that case.

Lymphoma usually appears as a bulky soft tissue mass associated with bone remodeling and expansion, although aggressive bone erosion can be seen. Occasionally, the sinus ostium is obstructed, causing expansion of the involved sinus. Once it is advanced, sinonasal lymphoma can involve the infratemporal fossa, orbit, and cranial fossa. On MRI, lymphoma tends to have intermediate signal intensity on T2-weighted image with homogeneous contrast enhancement. One of the advantages of MRI for sinonasal tumor is to differentiate neoplasm from obstructed sinuses. Dural invasion or perineural extension to the skull base is better evaluated with contrast-enhanced MRI. Treatment is usually combined radiation and chemotherapy.

Differential diagnosis should include sinonasal malignancies, such as squamous cell carcinoma, adenoid cystic carcinoma, mucoepidermoid carcinoma, extramedullary plasmacytoma, leukemia, or fungus infection and granulomatous disease in the nasal cavity (Wegener's granulomatosis). Because the lesion is immediately accessible for biopsy, the main role of imaging study is to define the extent of the lesion.

SUGGESTED READINGS

Ratech H, Burke JS, Blayney DW, et al. A clinicopathologic study of malignant lymphomas of the nose, paranasal sinuses, and hard palate including lethal midline granuloma. *Cancer* 1989;64:2525–2531.

Wilder WH, Harner SG, Banks PM. Lymphoma of the nose and paranasal sinuses. *Arch Otolaryngol* 1983;109:310–312.

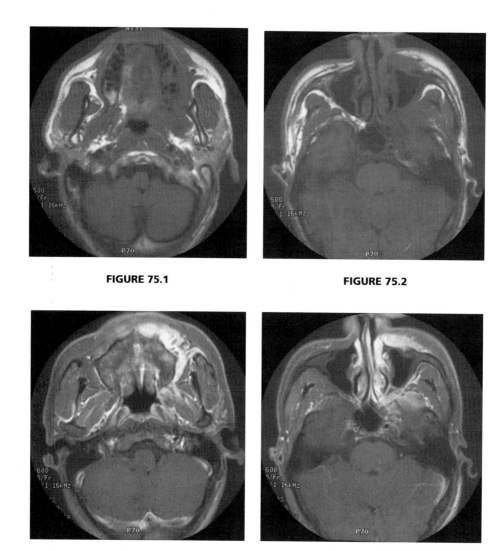

FIGURE 75.1

FIGURE 75.2

FIGURE 75.3

FIGURE 75.4

CLINICAL HISTORY

A 36-year-old man with a 7-month history of chronic maxillary pain and swelling undergoes treatment with antibiotics. He had a screening sinus CT scan 6 months previously, which did not show any abnormality. He presents with loosening of his maxillary incisors. He undergoes extraction of incisors and biopsy.

FINDINGS

T1-weighted axial images show an infiltrative mass extending from the lateral and posterior walls of the left maxillary sinus into the premalar region (Figs. 75.1, 75.2). Contrast-enhanced fat-suppressed image clearly shows a soft tissue mass in the masticator space and abnormal contrast enhancement extending to the superior orbital fissure via the pterygopalatine fossa (Figs. 75.3, 75.4).

DIAGNOSIS

Maxillary sinus squamous cell carcinoma with skull base invasion.

DISCUSSION

Squamous cell carcinoma is the most common sinonasal malignant tumor. Most cases of carcinoma of the maxillary sinuses are diagnosed only at an advanced stage. The prognosis is often poor because of the uncontrolled growth of the primary tumor. Cervical lymph node metastasis is uncommon. Imaging studies play an important role in defining the extent of tumor for staging. The staging of maxillary sinus cancer is based on Ohngren's line (from the medial canthus of the eye to the angle of the mandible), separating anteroinferior structures from superoposterior structures. It is crucial to identify whether the lesion invades the hard palate, floor or medial wall of the orbit, skin of the cheek, cribriform plate, nasopharynx, pterygomaxillary fossa, or posterior ethmoid or sphenoid sinuses.

CT is an excellent way to detect bone erosion or destruction. On CT, sinus malignancies often have a thickened enhancing mucosa associated with focal bone erosion. An early maxillary sinus carcinoma that is confined to the mucosa without bone erosion or destruction (T1 lesion on TNM classification), however, cannot be differentiated from sinus inflammatory disease on CT. When a screening sinus CT is used instead of a diagnostic sinus CT series for a patient with nonspecific facial pain such as in this case, subtle bone erosion may not be detected because of thick slice section and interslice gap. The other drawback of CT is its inability to differentiate tumor from inflammatory changes in the sinus when the two coexist in the same patient.

Unlike CT, MRI allows better differentiation of neoplasm from postobstructive fluid accumulations, because sinonasal malignancies tend to have lower T2 signal with respect to fluid collections within the paranasal sinuses. Exceptions occur with some minor salivary gland tumors and some neuromas that have bright signal on T2-weighted images. Tumors tend to have homogeneous contrast enhancement as opposed to rim enhancement seen with inflammatory mucosa. MRI also reveals the presence of perineural spread of neoplasm as seen in this case (tumor spread along V2 nerve which was confirmed at surgery).

The differential diagnosis in this case includes the following: (a) other primary maxillary sinus malignancies including squamous cell carcinoma, adenoid cystic carcinoma, melanoma, rhabdomyosarcoma, chondrosarcoma, osteogenic sarcoma, and lymphoma, (b) secondary tumors from the oral cavity or alveolar ridge, (c) metastases to the paranasal sinuses originating from the kidney, breast, lung, or gastrointestinal tract, (d) aggressive fungal infections that can produce both bone destruction and mass mimicking malignant tumors.

SUGGESTED READINGS

Dillon WP. Applications of magnetic resonance imaging to the head and neck. *Semin Ultrasound CT MR* 1986;7:202–215.

Mancuso AA, Hanafee WN. *Computed tomography and magnetic resonance imaging of the head and neck,* 2nd ed. Baltimore: Williams and Wilkins, 1985;4–7.

Som PM, Dillon WP, Sze G, et al. Benign and malignant sinonasal lesions with intracranial extension: differentiation with MR imaging. *Radiology* 1989;172:763–766.

Som PM, Shapiro MD, Biller HF, et al. Sinonasal tumors and inflammatory tissues: differentiation with MR imaging. *Radiology* 1988;167:803–808.

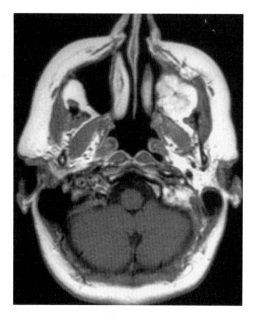

FIGURE 76.1

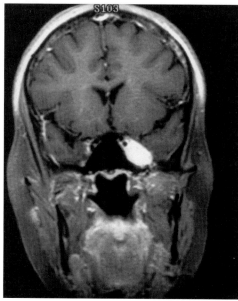

FIGURE 76.2

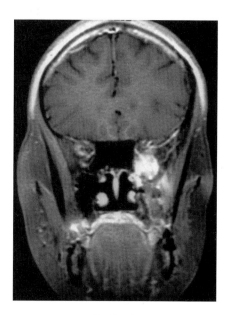

FIGURE 76.3

CLINICAL HISTORY

A 43-year-old woman presents with headache and hyperesthesia along V2 nerve.

FINDINGS

Postcontrast T1-weighted image shows a well-defined homogeneously enhancing mass in the left cavernous sinus with extension to the foramen rotundum and pterygopalatine fossa (Figs. 76.1, 76.2). The lower image shows a mass in the anterior masticator space and the posterior maxillary sinus (Fig. 76.3).

DIAGNOSIS

Hemangiopericytoma.

DISCUSSION

Hemangiopericytomas are slow-growing vascular neoplasms that arise from the pericytes of Zimmermann. They are composed of scattered capillary-like spaces surrounded by proliferating pericytes. They primarily affect extremities, retroperitoneum, and pelvis. Approximately 15% of tumors arise in the head and neck. They occur in the periorbital soft tissue, neck, and sinonasal cavity. The lesions are locally aggressive and often recur if not completely excised.

MRI shows a fairly well-defined mass with marked homogeneous contrast enhancement. CT may demonstrate focal bone erosion and remodeling associated with the tumor. On imaging studies, hemangiopericytoma cannot reliably be differentiated from meningioma, and other vascular tumors, such as angioleiomyoma, hemangioendothelioma, or malignant fibrous histiocytoma.

SUGGESTED READINGS

Enzinger FM, Smith BH. Hemangiopericytoma: an analysis of 106 cases. *Hum Pathol* 1976;7:61–82.
Staut AP, Murray MR. Hemangiopericytoma. *Ann Surg* 1972:116:26–32.

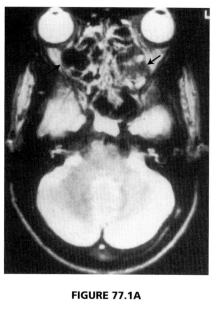

FIGURE 77.1A

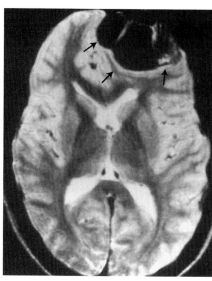

FIGURE 77.1B

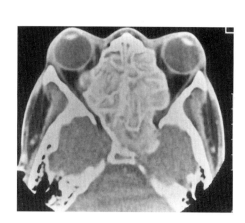

FIGURE 77.1C

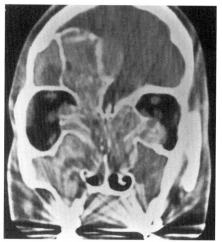

FIGURE 77.1D

CLINICAL HISTORY

A 24-year-old man presents with a history of rhinopolyposis and increasing headaches and proptosis.

FINDINGS

Axial T2-weighted MR study shows mixed signal intensities within the nasal vault and sinus cavities as a result of the different components present in this lesion (Fig. 77.1A). The frontal sinuses show a mass indenting the brain with a predominantly hypointense component with signal voids consistent with desiccated secretions (Fig. 77.1B). These signal voids may simulate aerated sinuses on MRI. CT of the paranasal sinuses shows extensive soft tissue masses involving the ethmoid, frontal, sphenoid, and maxillary sinuses. The axial view shows marked expansion of the ethmoid air cells bilaterally with demineralization and bowing of the medial wall of both orbits (Fig. 77.1C). There is orbital invasion causing bilateral proptosis. Posteriorly, this mass extends intracranially and invades the left cavernous sinus. On the coronal view, the intracranial extension to the left frontal region and intraorbital extension are better appreciated (Fig. 77.1D). These CT and MR patterns, although showing some aggressive features that could suggest a malignant neoplastic condition, are more characteristic of a benign process.

In particular, note the integrity of the bony trabecula in the ethmoid sinus and the presence of a hypodense rim separating the central hyperdense soft tissue mass from the sinus walls on the CT images and the mixed signal intensities seen on the MR study. (Images courtesy of Dr. Peter Som.)

DIAGNOSIS

Mucocele formation in the ethmoid, frontal, and sphenoid sinuses in a patient with rhinopolyposis.

DISCUSSION

Mucoceles result from obstruction of the ostium of a sinus cavity, leading to progressive accumulation of the secretions trapped within the sinus. Retention cysts, which result from obstruction of the duct of a single mucous gland, can be potentially indistinguishible from a mucocele if large enough to fill the sinus. However, retention cysts do not usually grow large enough to cause expansion of a sinus cavity. Retention cysts are lined by the epithelium of the obstructed gland and are a frequent finding in patients referred for radiologic studies of the paranasal sinus (up to 10% in some series).

The most common mechanism of obstruction preventing sinus drainage is chronic inflammation resulting in thickening of the mucosa of the paranasal ostium or from chronic nasal polyposis. Other causes that can lead to obstruction include congenital anomalies, trauma, prior sinus surgery, fibro-osseous lesions, neoplasia, and diseases associated with viscid inspissated secretions such as cystic fibrosis. Mucoceles are rare in the pediatric population. When present in this age group, cystic fibrosis should be considered. The presence of complete bony septations within sinus cavity can isolate a compartment within the sinus and is associated with an increased risk of mucocele formation.

Several hypotheses have been proposed to explain the expansile nature of this lesion. A combination of pressure necrosis, bone devascularization, and release of osteolytic enzymes appear to be the most important factors in the pathogenesis of mucoceles. Osteolysis of the inner table of the sinus cavity is accompanied by periosteal new bone formation of the outer table, leading to remodeling and subsequent expansion. When bone destruction overcomes bone formation, there is destruction of the bony sinus wall and the mucocele is bounded only by its own mucosal lining.

Mucoceles are far more frequent in the frontal sinus (60%) because of the small caliber, tortuosity, and long course of the nasofrontal duct. Ethmoid (30%), maxillary (10%), and sphenoid (<1%) follow in order of decreasing frequency.

Symptoms depend on the location of the mucocele and result either from mechanical effects or superinfection. Mass effects include bossing of the forehead, nasal vault, or cheek, nasal obstruction, proptosis, headaches, orbital apex syndrome, and cranial nerve palsies. When infected, mucoceles are known as mucopyoceles, and may cause pain and systemic symptoms.

The most frequent complications of mucoceles are orbital and intracranial invasion and infection. Intraorbital invasion with optic nerve impingement can result in irreversible visual loss. For this reason, mucoceles should always be considered in the differential diagnosis in a patient with sudden onset of visual loss. Other cranial nerve palsies can occur, especially in sphenoid sinus mucoceles extending laterally into the cavernous sinus. Chronic dural inflammation may be responsible for some cranial nerve palsies when direct mechanical compression of the cranial nerves is not documented. Meningitis is another possible complication when infection of the mucocele occurs (mucopyocele).

Mucoceles can be diagnosed on plain films of the paranasal sinus, but CT and MRI are superior in defining the extension and potential complications of this condition and are essential for therapy planning.

CT is the ideal method to evaluate the bony changes and integrity of the bony margins of the sinus walls. CT discloses an expansile nonenhancing mass filling a sinus cavity. The density of this mass depends on the chronicity of the lesion and composition of the retained secretions.

MRI is the best tool to depict intraorbital and intracranial extension and is helpful in the differential diagnosis from malignancy when contrast material is used. The signal characteristics depend on the protein and water content of the secretions and several patterns can be seen. In the early stages, watery mucous secretions show hypointensity on T1-weighted and hyperintensity on T2-weighted images. Desiccated stagnant secretions may show low signal on both T1- and T2-weighted images. With paramagnetic contrast administration, mucoceles enhance peripherally even when not infected but never centrally as do most neoplasms.

The presence of signal void within a sinus on both T1- and T2-weighted images can represent a variety of conditions including a normal aerated sinus, desiccated secretions, calcifications, fungal concretions (mycetoma), foreign body, ectopic tooth, dentigerous cyst, and fresh blood. Care must be taken not to misdiagnose a mucocele filled with desiccated secretions for a normal aerated sinus. One should always look for signs of expansion or perform CT in doubtful cases. When infection is present and complicated by meningitis, dural enhancement can also be depicted with both CT and MR.

Even when asymptomatic, mucoceles are usually treated because they behave like slow-growing neoplasms and are potentially life threatening. Two different approaches can be used: intranasal endoscopic surgery or open obliterative surgery.

Intranasal endoscopic treatment is the modality of choice for ethmoid and sphenoid sinus mucoceles, especially when intracranial or intraorbital extension is present. Frontal sinus mucoceles have been treated using a limited frontal craniotomy, removal of the mucocele and all mucosa, followed by stripping of the mucosa and packing the sinus with fat tissue (Lynch procedure or osteoplastic flap). Recent work has shown some advantage to using endoscopic surgery in frontal sinus mucoceles, whether or not intracranial or intraorbital extension is present.

The main goal of therapy is to achieve decompression of the mucocele in order to relieve the symptoms associated with mass effect. Several advantages of the endoscopic technique have been documented. This technique can be performed on an outpatient basis, sometimes under local anesthesia, with no external incisions required and a lower rate of complications such as cerebrospinal fluid leaks and meningitis in comparison with the open obliterative procedure. Imaging follow-up is recommended in every case to check for recurrence.

SUGGESTED READINGS

Benninger MS, Marks S. The endoscopic management of sphenoid and ethmoid mucoceles with orbital and intranasal extension. *Rhinology* 1995;33:157–161.

Chua R, Shapiro S. A mucopyocele of the clivus: case report. *Neurosurgery* 1996;39:589–590; discussion 590–591.

Delfini R, Missori P, Iannetti G, et al. Mucoceles of the paranasal sinuses with intracranial and intraorbital extension: report of 28 cases. *Neurosurgery* 1993;32:901–906; discussion 906.

Fligny I, Lamas G, Aidan P, et al. Frontal mucocele. Clinical symptoms, treatment and results apropos of 17 cases. *Acta Otorhinolaryngol Belg* 1993;47:429–434.

Gentile VG, Isaacson G. Patterns of sinusitis in cystic fibrosis. *Laryngoscope* 1996;106:1005–1009.

Har-el G. Telescopic extracranial approach to frontal mucoceles with intracranial extension. *J Otolaryngol* 1995;24:98–101.

Kemissi E, Balo K, Kpodzro K. Sinus mucoceles. Apropos of 5 cases. *Ann Otolaryngol Chir Cervicofaciale* 1996;113:179–182.

Krishnan G, Kumar G. Frontoethmoid mucocele: one-year follow-up after endoscopic frontoethmoidectomy. *J Otolaryngol* 1996;25:37–40.

Selvapandian S, Rajshekhar V, Chandy MJ. Mucoceles: a neurosurgical perspective. *Br J Neurosurg* 1994;8:57–61.

Sterling KM, Stollman A, Sacher M, et al. Ossifying fibroma of sphenoid bone with coexistent mucocele: CT and MRI. *J Comput Assist Tomogr* 1993;17:492–494.

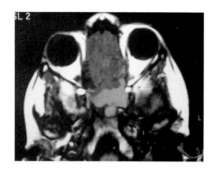

FIGURE 78.1A

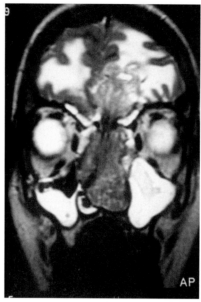

FIGURE 78.1B

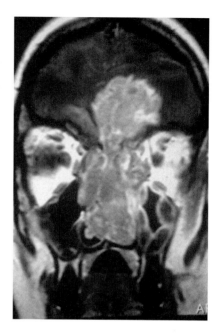

FIGURE 78.1C

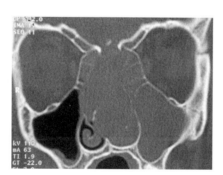

FIGURE 78.1D

CLINICAL HISTORY

A 17-year-old female presents with nasal obstruction and epistaxis.

FINDINGS

Axial T1-weighted, coronal T2-weighted, contrast-enhanced coronal T1-weighted, and coronal CT section through the paranasal sinuses (Fig. 78.1A–D) show a large nasoethmoidal mass with intracranial and bilateral extraconal orbital invasion. There is extensive destruction of the cribriform plate best seen on the coronal CT image (Fig. 78.1D) and bilateral erosion of the posterior aspect of the lamina papyracea. The mass fills in most of the nasal cavity, more prominently on the left side, bowing the nasal septum to the right. There is a large intracranial component in the anterior cranial fossa with prominent edema of the frontal lobes. Postobstructive changes are noted in the frontal, sphenoid, and maxillary sinuses. The lesion is heterogeneous on the T2-weighted images, showing small areas of necrosis and cystic degeneration in the intracranial portion.

DIAGNOSIS

Esthesioneuroblastoma.

DISCUSSION

Esthesioneuroblastomas, or olfactory neuroblastomas, are neural crest tumors that arise from neuroectodermal stem cells lining the cribriform plate and nasal vault. These malignant tumors are locally aggressive, tend to recur locally, and have a 20% rate of hematogenous metastases, most commonly to cervical lymph nodes, lung, liver, bone, and brain. Staging systems based on tumor extension are useful in treatment planning and determining prognosis. These include the Kaddish-Goodman and Wine and the TNM systems. The most commonly used is the TNM system recently modified by Biller in which the primary tumor is subdivided in four grades: T1 when the tumor is limited to the sinonasal cavities with or without cribriform plate erosion, T2 when there is intracranial extension without brain invasion, T3 when resectable brain invasion is present, and T4 when there is unresectable brain or skull base invasion.

There is a bimodal distribution with incidence peaks in the second and sixth decades. Patients present with nonspecific sinonasal complaints including nasal stuffiness, nasal discharge, and epistaxis, which are often mistaken for inflammatory conditions such as chronic rhinosinusitis or nasal polyposis. Anosmia is a frequent finding and is due to tumor location in the olfactory epithelium. Headaches, facial pain, and proptosis are symptoms associated with larger tumors that have already transgressed the bony boundaries of the sinonasal region. On rhinoscopy, these tumors are fleshy and may have a polypoid appearance, sometimes mimicking inflammatory polyps. Because of their rich vascularity, they bleed easily during the examination and after biopsy.

Cross-sectional imaging is mandatory, both in the diagnosis and staging. Although imaging findings are nonspecific, both on CT and MRI, all sinonasal masses associated with bony destruction or spread beyond the sinonasal region should be viewed with suspicion and correlated with rhinoscopy findings and biopsy. CT is the best modality to detect bony remodeling, thinning, or erosion of the cribriform plate, lamina papyracea, nasal septum, and nasal turbinates and to detect tumor calcifications. On the other hand, MRI is valuable to evaluate tumor extension because it separates neoplastic tissue from inflammatory postobstructive changes and adequately depicts any intraorbital or intracranial spread. Clues to the diagnosis include location in the nasal vault and anterior ethmoid region, intermediate signal intensity on T2-weighted images typical of highly cellular tumors, and the presence of small cysts at the periphery of the tumor.

Other small cell tumors such as lymphoma share similar signal characteristics. Vivid enhancement is seen on both CT and MRI and is useful to delineate any intracranial and intraorbital components. Tumor spread occurs superiorly to anterior cranial fossa, through the cribriform plate, laterally into the orbits after transgressing the lamina papyracea, and downward into the nasal cavity and other perinasal cavities. Although conventional angiography is not part of the imaging protocol for these tumors, it shows an intense vascular blush in the nasoethmoidal region.

Differential diagnosis includes other sinonasal malignancies (squamous cell carcinoma, adenocarcinoma, minor salivary gland tumors, lymphoma, melanoma, and sarcomas), some benign tumors (inverted papilloma and olfactory groove meningioma, among others), and aggressive infectious processes and inflammatory conditions, particularly mucoceles. All these conditions may present on imaging studies as masses that remodel or erode bone.

Surgical resection is the treatment of choice. Since it was proven that microscopic disease, mainly in the cribriform plate, is responsible for most recurrences, extensive surgeries using wide craniofacial resections and postoperative radiation therapy have been advocated. Chemotherapy has also been advised for high-grade tumors and when there are positive tumor margins. Using these combined therapies, 5-year survival rates have increased to 92%.

SUGGESTED READINGS

Derdeyn CP, Moran CJ, Wippold FJ 2nd, et al. MRI of esthesioneuroblastoma. *J Comput Assist Tomogr* 1994;18:16–21.

Eustace S, Suojanen J, Buff B, et al. Preoperative imaging of esthesioneuroblastoma. *Clin Radiol* 1995;59:639–643.

Li C, Yoseum DM, Hayden RE, et al. Olfactory neuroblastoma: MR evaluation. *AJNR Am J Neuroradiol* 1993;14:1167–1171.

Slevin NJ, Irwin CJ, Banerjee SS, et al. Olfactory neural tumors: the role of external beam radiation therapy. *J Laryngol Otol* 1996;110:1012–1016.

Woodhead P, Loyd GA. Olfactory neuroblastoma: imaging by magnetic resonance, CT and conventional techniques. *Clin Otolaryngol* 1998;13:387–394.

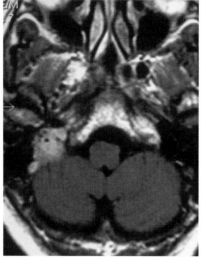

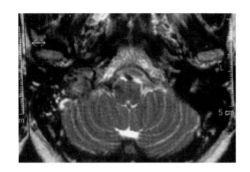

FIGURE 79.1A

FIGURE 79.1B

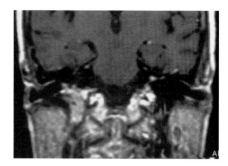

FIGURE 79.1C

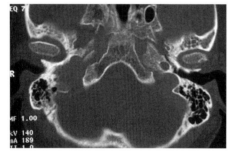

FIGURE 79.2

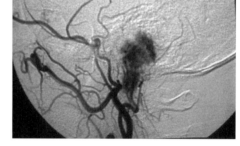

FIGURE 79.3

CLINICAL HISTORY

A 45-year-old woman presents with pulsatile tinnitus.

FINDINGS

There is a large lesion centered in the right jugular foramen extending anteriorly into the middle ear cavity in the region of the hypotympanum. The mass is heterogeneous with areas of hyperintensity and serpiginous hypointensities seen on the axial T2-weighted image (Fig. 79.1A) with a "salt and pepper" pattern and enhances vividly on both the axial and coronal T1-weighted postgadolinium images (Fig. 79.1B, C). CT axial section through the jugular foramen demonstrates erosion of the jugular spine and caroticojugular crest (Fig. 79.2). A conventional angiogram shows a large hypervascular mass supplied by external carotid artery branches (Fig. 79.3).

DIAGNOSIS

Glomus jugulotympanicum.

DISCUSSION

Glomus tumors or paragangliomas are benign slow-growing tumors that arise from glomus bodies. These glomus bodies are embryologic derivatives of the neural crest and belong to the diffuse neuroendocrine system scattered along some cranial nerves. In the temporal bone region, they are located along the tympanic branch of cranial nerve IX and the auricular branch of cranial nerve X, known by the eponyms of Jacobsen's and Arnold's nerves. Both these branches run along the adventitia of the jugular vein before entering the temporal bone. Based on their location within the temporal bone, they are classified into three subtypes: glomus jugulare, in which the tumor is confined to the jugular foramen; glomus tympanicum, in which the tumor is limited to the middle ear cavity; and glomus jugulotympanicum, in which the tumor involves both the jugular foramen and middle ear cavity. This division has major implications in surgical management.

Similarly to paragangliomas arising from other sites, glomus jugulotympanicum tumors have specific imaging features. They are highly vascular tumors showing vivid contrast enhancement on both MRI and CT imaging, and they usually have well-defined borders. Because most tumors are benign and slow growing, they begin to enlarge and remodel the jugular foramen and to grow along paths of least resistance, burrowing into fissures, grooves, and natural foramina. When large enough, they erode the jugular spine and the caroticojugular crest, and may grow anteriorly through the jugular plate into the middle ear cavity, following the course of Jacobsen's nerve along the inferior tympanic canaliculus. CT is the best imaging modality to demonstrate subtle bony erosion, which is crucial in the differential diagnosis between glomus jugulare and vascular anomalies, such as high-riding or dehiscent jugular bulb. Besides the diagnostic role, conventional angiography may detect small synchronous tumors and is performed with the goal of preoperative embolization. This procedure dramatically reduces the surgical morbidity related to bleeding. Arterial supply is most frequently derived from external carotid branches of the ascending pharyngeal, internal maxillary, stylomastoid, and occipital arteries. Supply from the petrous internal carotid artery via caroticotympanic branches is also seen, particularly in large tumors.

The most common other pathologic processes arising within or in the vicinity of the jugular foramen include schwannomas of cranial nerves IX to XII, meningiomas, sarcomas, metastases, and invasion from nasopharyngeal carcinomas.

Paragangliomas have a higher incidence in women and in persons between the fourth and sixth decades of life. The 10% rule states that 10% of paragangliomas are familial (autosomal dominant pattern of inheritance), 10% of nonfamilial cases are multifocal, and 10% are associated with malignant tumors in other organs. Multifocality in familial cases has an incidence of 30%. Malignant degeneration and metastasis are seen in 4% of cases.

Presenting symptoms depend on tumor size and location. Most commonly, jugulotympanic paragangliomas present either with otologic or cranial nerve symptoms (Vernet's syndrome). These include pulsatile tinnitus, conductive hearing loss, and lower cranial nerve deficits. Facial nerve palsy may ensue when the tumor extends to involve the mastoid or tympanic segments of the facial nerve. A minority of secreting tumors (3%) present with neuroendocrinologic symptoms.

Most glomus jugulotympanicum tumors are managed surgically after embolization of their major arterial supply. When surgery is contraindicated, tumor control may be achieved with radiation therapy.

SUGGESTED READINGS

Baguley DM, Irving RM, Hardy DG, et al. Audiologic findings in the evaluation of glomus tympanicum tumors. *Br J Audiol* 1994;28:291–297.

LaRouere MJ, Zappia JJ, Wilner HI. Selective embolization of glomus jugulare tumors. Skill base surgery. 1994;4:21–25.

Vogl T, Bruning R, Schedel H. Paragangliomas of the jugular bulb and carotid body; MR imaging with short sequences and GD-DTPA enhancement. *AJNR Am J Neuroradiol* 1989;10:823–827.

Weber AL, Mckenna NJ. Radiologic evaluation of the jugular foramen, vascular variants, anomalies and tumors. *Neuroimaging Clin North Am* 1994;4:579–598.

Weissman JL, Hirsh BE. Beyond the promontory: the multifocal origin of glomus tympanicum tumors. *AJNR Am J Neuroradiol* 1998;19:119–122.

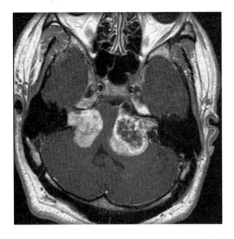

FIGURE 80.1A

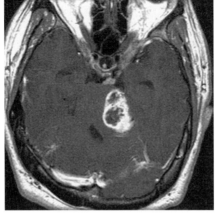

FIGURE 80.1B

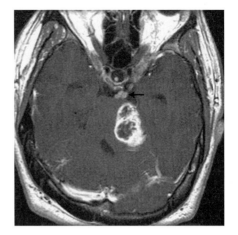

FIGURE 80.1C

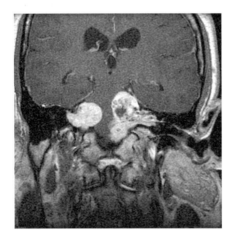

FIGURE 80.1D

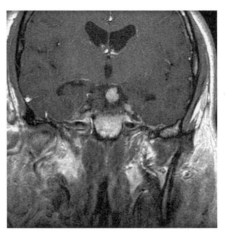

FIGURE 80.1E

CLINICAL HISTORY

A 35-year-old man presents with bilateral sensorineural hearing loss. He has a history of radiosurgery for brain tumors.

FINDINGS

Axial T1-weighted enhanced MRI of the brain shows bilateral enhancing CPA tumors with intra-canalicular components with severe brainstem distortion (Fig. 80.1A). The central portion of the left mass shows areas of nonenhancement (Fig. 80.1B). The higher section shows an enhancing mass in the region of the third nerve (Fig. 80.1C). Coronal T1-weighted enhanced views again show the CPA masses (Fig. 80.1D). The third nerve mass is seen in the more anterior view (Fig. 80.1E).

DIAGNOSIS

Neurofibromatosis type II (NFII) presenting with bilateral vestibular schwannomas and left oculomotor schwannoma.

DISCUSSION

NFII is the second most common phakomatosis following NFI. It has an estimated incidence of 1:50,000 people in the general population. More than 50% of patients present before 25 years of age with bilateral sensorineural hearing loss; 10% become symptomatic before age 10 years.

NFII is a genetic disorder with a high degree of penetrance that may be inherited as an autosomal dominant trait or acquired by spontaneous mutation. The NFII gene has been localized in the 12 locus of the long arm of chromosome 22 (22q12). This gene encodes for a protein named *merlin* or *schwannomin,* which acts as a tumor suppressor. Different mutations in this gene have been identified, leading to different abnormalities in the protein product. These different mutations not only correlate with different degrees in the severity of NFII but are also responsible for NFII variants such as schwannomatosis, NFII mosaicism (segmental NFII), and multiple meningiomas. Abnormalities in the 22q12 gene locus are associated with NFII as well as being present in patients with unilateral vestibular schwannomas, meningiomas, and other neoplasms, such as melanoma, breast carcinoma, and malignant mesothelioma.

The diagnosis of NFII is still made clinically because a cost-effective genetic test for mutation detection has not yet been created. Nearly all patients with NFII present with sensorineural hearing loss, most before age 25 years. Other signs and symptoms depend on the location of other tumors in the peripheral or central nervous system. Definite diagnosis of NFII is made in the presence of bilateral vestibular schwannomas or family history of NFII in a first degree relative plus unilateral vestibular schwannoma before age 30 or any two of the following: meningioma, glioma, schwannoma, juvenile posterior subcapsular lenticular opacity, or juvenile cortical cataract. Evaluation for NFII must include long-term follow-up and a single evaluation is inadequate.

Patients with a family history of NFII, with unilateral vestibular schwannoma or meningioma before age 30, or with multiple spinal tumors are at risk for NFII (presumptive or probable NFII) and should be further evaluated. The diagnosis of presumptive NFII includes unilateral vestibular schwannoma before age 30 plus one of the following: meningioma, glioma, schwannoma, juvenile posterior subcapsular lenticular opacity, juvenile cortical cataract, or two or more meningiomas plus unilateral vestibular schwannoma before age 30 or one of the following: glioma, schwannoma, juvenile posterior subcapsular lenticular opacity, or juvenile cortical cataract.

The imaging modality of choice both for screening and follow-up of patients with NFII is MRI. It provides optimal depiction of all the central nervous system tumors commonly seen in NFII including schwannomas, meningiomas, ependymomas, and occasional gliomas or neurofibromas. Following cranial nerve VIII, the trigeminal nerve is the second most common site for schwannomas in NFII. Care should be taken to avoid confusion between dural ectasia of the nerve sheath, causing flaring of the IAC, and vestibular schwannoma. The former follows the signal intensity of cerebrospinal fluid and does not show contrast enhancement. Meningiomas are the second most common tumor type seen in patients with NFII. Meningiomatosis, characterized by innumerable small meningiomas seeding the dura, may occur in the setting of definitive NFII or as an NFII variant.

The treatment of NFII is based on surgical treatment of the neoplasms associated with the disease. The major problem in patients with NFII is bilateral sensorineural hearing loss leading to deafness at an early age. Decisions regarding conservative surgical or radiosurgical therapy of vestibular schwannomas are complex and controversial, especially in this new era of brainstem implants. Small, less than 1.5-cm vestibular schwannomas confined to the IAC can often be completely resected with preservation of hearing and facial nerve function. Stereotactic radiosurgery or gamma knife radiosurgery may be used as an alternative to surgery or as neoadjuvant therapy for residual disease. This modality may lead to regression in tumor size or arrest in tumor growth, but it is not devoid of complications. Other brain and spinal tumors such as meningiomas, other cranial nerve schwannomas, and ependymomas should be closely monitored for growth and imaged symptomatically.

SUGGESTED READINGS

Bikhazi NB, Slattery WH 3rd, Lalwani AK, et al. Familial occurrence of unilateral vestibular schwannoma. *Laryngoscope* 1997;107:1176–1180.

Deen HG, Ebersold MJ, Harner SG, et al. Conservative management of acoustic neuroma: an outcome study. *Neurosurgery* 1996;39:260–264; discussion 264–266.

Evans DG, Ramsden R, Huson SM, et al. Type 2 neurofibromatosis: the need for supraregional care? *J Laryngol Otol* 1993;107:401–406.

Gutmann DH, Aylsworth A, Carey JC, et al. The diagnostic evaluation and multidisciplinary management of neurofibromatosis 1 and neurofibromatosis 2. *JAMA* 1997;278:51–57.

Val-Bernal JF, Figols J, Vázquez-Barquero A. Cutaneous plexiform schwannoma associated with neurofibromatosis type 2. *Cancer* 1995;76:1181–1186.

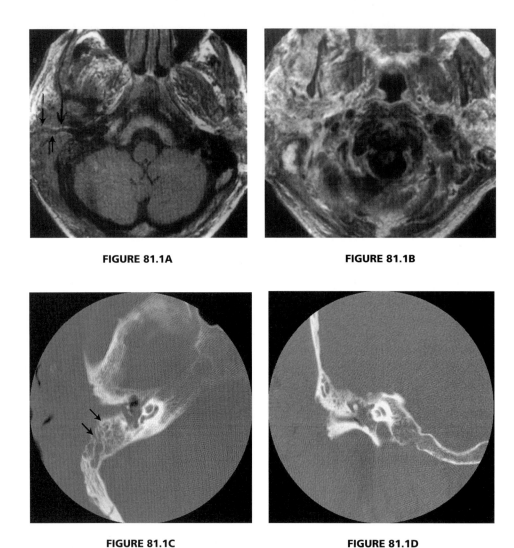

FIGURE 81.1A

FIGURE 81.1B

FIGURE 81.1C

FIGURE 81.1D

CLINICAL HISTORY

A 64-year-old diabetic man presents with a 2-week history of right-sided otorrhea and otalgia unresponsive to antibiotics. Four days before presentation, he noted right cheek swelling and trismus.

FINDINGS

Axial T1-weighted MRI of the temporal bones and neck shows marked swelling and abnormal soft tissue thickening in the external auditory canal on the right, obliterating the fascial planes (Fig. 81.1A). Soft tissue swelling is also noted along the lateral aspect of the mastoid bone and temporal squamosa, extending posteriorly to the occipital region. There is opacification of most mastoid air cells and in the re-

gion of the middle ear cleft. This abnormal soft tissue shows intense enhancement on the postcontrast image (Fig. 81.1B). The right masseter and lateral pterygoid muscles are enlarged and markedly enhanced. The lateral cortical margin of the mastoid bone appears disrupted.

Axial CT of the temporal bones was performed to further characterize the bony changes and shows cortical erosion and disruption of the posterior wall of the bony external auditory canal (EAC) and cortical margin of the lateral wall of the right mastoid (Fig. 81.1C). There is abnormal soft tissue density in the right EAC and partial opacification of the right middle ear cavity. Most of the mastoid air cells are opacified. The ossicular chain is neither displaced nor eroded. The coronal view confirms these findings (Fig. 81.1D).

DIAGNOSIS

Malignant otitis externa.

DISCUSSION

Malignant external otitis is a severe infectious process that begins in the EAC and frequently spreads throughout the temporal bone, skull base, and suprahyoid neck, crossing fascial planes. Other terms commonly used to refer to this entity are *necrotizing* or *invasive otitis externa.* It is a rare entity, typically presenting in elderly diabetic patients. However, it may be seen with other forms of immunosuppression, as in acquired immunodeficiency syndrome, in which the disease may present in younger patients.

The most common agent is *Pseudomonas aeruginosa,* an opportunistic organism that tends to grow in moist environments and devitalized tissues, especially when there is an imbalance in the normal commensal flora. Less frequently, other agents have been implicated. Predisposing factors include diabetes mellitus, immunosuppression (congenital or acquired), history of prior EAC lavage, and chronic use of antimicrobial agents that do not cover *Pseudomonas* species.

The inciting event appears to be a dermatitis of the EAC, compromising the normal barrier of the skin. This may be due to trauma after syringe jet lavage or repeated introduction of foreign bodies into the EAC. In diabetic patients, microangiopathy resulting from endarteritis may compromise the microcirculation in the EAC, increasing the susceptibility to infection (ischemic perichondritis). The moist environment of the EAC, especially after repeated use of topical antibiotics to cover other agents of otitis externa, further favors the growth of the commensal *P. aeruginosa.*

The infection usually begins at the junction of the cartilaginous and bony portions of the EAC and from there spreads insidiously and silently to the temporal bone and surrounding structures.

The pattern of spread is fairly consistent. Initially, the disease tends to spread inferiorly, through the small clefts normally present in the floor of the EAC (fissures of Santorini), to involve the soft tissues inferior to the temporal bone, including the parotid space, infratemporal masticator space, and skull base. Less common routes of dissemination include posterior spread to the mastoid air cells, anterior spread into the temporomandibular joint (TMJ), and medial spread into the middle ear cavity and petrous apex.

The most common presenting symptoms are unrelenting otalgia and purulent otorrhea despite antibiotic therapy. This purulent otorrhea, may be scant or profuse and typically presents as a foul-smelling greenish exudate. With disease progression, headaches, usually located over the temporal bone region, pain in the TMJ, trismus, and cranial nerve palsies may ensue. The presence of headaches and cranial nerve palsies usually indicate skull base osteomyelitis. Trismus results from involvement of the TMJ or nasopharyngeal masticator space. The cranial nerve most commonly affected is the facial nerve resulting from progression of infection through the stylomastoid foramen or direct involvement of the facial nerve canal in the tympanic or mastoid segments.

The major goals of imaging are to determine disease extent, identify drainable fluid collections, evaluate the success of therapy, and help confirm the diagnosis.

CT is the modality of choice, because it adequately depicts cortical bony changes, which, when present, are the hallmark of this disease. MRI is used as an adjunct to evaluate the soft tissue extent and detect any intracranial complications. MRI may also detect bone marrow changes in the skull base, which may not be apparent on CT.

Osteolysis may never resolve after complete eradication of the disease.

The most common CT finding is the presence of a soft tissue density in the EAC. However, this finding lacks specificity because it may represent a variety of pathologic entities. The presence of bony erosion and cortical disruption of the bony EAC, mastoid, or skull base in conjunction with a concordant clinical history is the hallmark of this entity. CT may also demonstrate opacification of the middle ear cavity and mastoid air cells resulting from postobstructive changes or direct extension of granulation tissue. Soft tissue changes include obliteration of the fascial and fat planes, initially beneath the EAC and later involving the parotid, parapharyngeal, and masticator spaces.

On MRI, the soft tissue changes may be better delineated. The inflammatory tissue in malignant external otitis is nonspecific in appearance (isointense to muscle on T1-weighted image and hyperintense on T2-weighted image), showing intense enhancement except in areas of tissue necrosis. However, some studies describe this inflammatory tissue as hypointense on both T1- and T2-weighted images, with scant enhancement. These features are thought to indicate the denser nature of this soft tissue material and its tendency to fibrose.

Precontrast and postcontrast images should always be obtained to allow detection of bone marrow changes and meningeal enhancement. Fat-suppressed images may be helpful in selected cases, in which the abnormal soft tissue is surrounded by fat.

Antibiotic therapy is the mainstay of treatment and should be directed to the etiologic agent. Because most cases are caused by *P. aeruginosa,* the treatment of choice is long term (6 to 8 weeks) ciprofloxacin. In extensive cases, a course of intravenous antibiotics may be warranted to halt progression. In the presence of osteomyelitis with bony sequestra or abscess formation, surgery should be performed with drainage and extensive debridement of the necrotic tissue.

SUGGESTED READINGS

Amorosa L, Modugno GC, Pirodda A. Malignant external otitis: review and personal experience. *Acta Otolaryngol Suppl* 1996;521:3–16.

Gordon G, Giddings NA. Invasive otitis externa due to *Aspergillus* species: case report and review. *Clin Infect Dis* 1994;19:866–870.

Grandis JR, Curtin HD, Yu VL. Necrotizing (malignant) external otitis: prospective comparison of CT and MR imaging in diagnosis and follow-up. *Radiology* 1995;196:499–504.

Hern JD, Almeyda J, Thomas DM, et al. Malignant otitis externa in HIV and AIDS. *J Laryngol Otol* 1996;110:770–775.

Hickham M, Amedee RG. Malignant otitis externa. *J Louisiana State Med Soc* 1996;148:511–513.

Lucente FE, Parisier SC, Chandler JR. Malignant external otitis. (*Laryngoscope* 1968;78:1257–1294). *Laryngoscope* 1996;106:805–807.

Manfrini S, Gregorio F, Capoolicasa E. Diabetes mellitus and malignant external otitis: a case study. *J Diabetes Complications* 1996;10:2–5.

Slattery WH 3rd, Brackmann DE. Skull base osteomyelitis. Malignant external otitis. *Otolaryngol Clin North Am* 1996;29:795–806.

Stokkel MP, Boot CN, van Eck-Smit BL. SPECT gallium scintigraphy in malignant external otitis: initial staging and follow-up. Case reports. *Laryngoscope* 1996;106(3 Pt 1):338–340.

Wormald PJ. Surgical management of benign necrotizing otitis externa. *J Laryngol Otol* 1994:108:101–105.

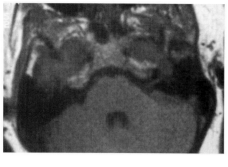

FIGURE 82.1A

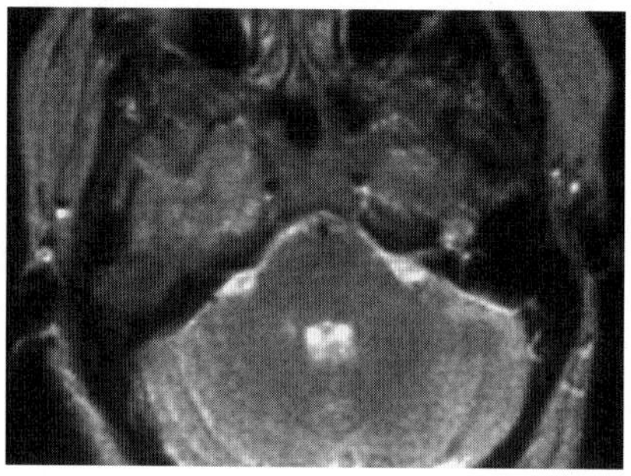

FIGURE 82.1B

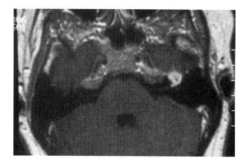

FIGURE 82.1C

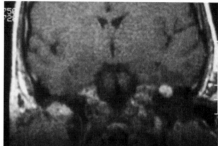

FIGURE 82.1D

CLINICAL HISTORY

A 37-year-old woman presents with facial nerve palsy and twitching.

FINDINGS

Axial T1- and T2-weighted and axial and coronal T1-weighted images after gadolinium administration (Fig. 82.1A–D) show a 10-mm mass along the labyrinthine segment of the left facial nerve with the major bulk of the mass in the region of the geniculate ganglion. The mass is isointense to brain on T1-weighted image and hyperintense on T2-weighted image, and enhances heterogeneously, showing a small central nonenhancing area. There is also linear enhancement in the porus acusticus.

DIAGNOSIS

Facial nerve schwannoma.

DISCUSSION

The incidence of facial nerve tumors in patients presenting with peripheral facial nerve palsy is rare, ranging from 6% to 10% according to different series. Among these, the most frequent are schwannomas, followed by hemangiomas, choristomas, lipomas, and paragangliomas. Most malignant neoplasms result from secondary perineural spread of sali-

vary gland malignancies, most commonly originating in the parotid gland.

Schwannomas are benign, slow-growing tumors resulting from abnormal proliferation of Schwann cells. They are composed of two different tissue types called Antoni A (compactly arranged spindle cells) and Antoni B (loosely arranged myxoid tissue, which may show cystic degeneration and hemorrhage). Schwannomas can occur anywhere along the course of the facial nerve but the most frequent location is the geniculate ganglion.

Clinical findings depend on tumor location. Tumors located in the geniculate ganglion and labyrinthine segment have a late presentation either with facial nerve symptoms (slow, progressive onset of facial nerve palsy associated with twitching) or compressive symptoms of the middle cranial fossa structures when the tumor grows anteriorly. Intracanalicular schwannomas tend to present with sensorineural hearing loss resulting from compression of the tightly packed, thinly myelinated fibers of the vestibulocochlear nerve, which is more vulnerable to compression and ischemia. Therefore, a tumor in this region may be difficult or impossible to differentiate from a vestibular schwannoma, both on clinical and imaging grounds.

Tumors involving the tympanic segment manifest with conductive hearing loss caused by the close relationships between the nerve, the oval window, and the ossicular chain. In the mastoid segment where the nerve is confined to a narrow bony canal, tumors may lead to sudden onset of facial nerve palsy, mimicking Bell's palsy. When the lesion extends or arises in the parotid segment, it may present as a parotid mass.

Imaging should be performed in all patients with slow onset, recurrent, or persistent (more than 3 months) facial nerve palsy or with facial nerve twitching. Facial nerve tumors present as a soft tissue mass along the course of the facial nerve. CT is helpful in depicting any abnormal enlargement, remodeling, or erosion of the facial nerve canal (fallopian canal). However, this finding is only present when the tumor becomes large enough to expand the surrounding bone. Small tumors may only be detected on MRI, which is also the best imaging modality to evaluate tumor extent. Most schwannomas are isointense to brain on T1-weighted images and hyperintense on T2-weighted images, and enhance homogeneously on postcontrast images. Large tumors tend to be more heterogeneous, showing areas of cystic or hemorrhagic transformation. Tumors of the geniculate ganglion may grow anteriorly into the middle cranial fossa and assume an hourglass shape.

Whenever a focal enhancing lesion is detected along the course of the facial nerve it is mandatory to include the parotid gland in the study to exclude the possibility of perineural spread of a salivary malignancy. Multifocal, linear, or nodular enhancement favors this possibility.

Treatment is surgical with end-to-end reconstruction of the facial nerve or, when the tumor is too extensive, with facial nerve grafting.

SUGGESTED READINGS

Chen JM, Moll C, Wichmann W, et al. Magnetic resonance imaging and intraoperative frozen sections in intratemporal facial schwannomas. *Am J Otol* 1995;16:68–74.

Fagan PA, Misra RN, Doust B. Facial neuroma of the cerebello-pontine angle and the internal auditory canal. *Laryngoscope* 1993;103:442–446.

Hajjaj M, Linthicum FH Jr. Facial nerve schwannoma: nerve fiber dissemination. *J Laryngol Otol* 1996;91:103–109.

Mcmenomey SO, Glasscock ME 3rd, Minor LB, et al. Facial nerve neuromas presenting as acoustic tumors. *Am J Otol* 1994;15:307–312.

Tew JM Jr, Yeh HS, Miller GW, et al. Intratemporal schwannoma of the facial nerve. *Neurosurgery* 1983;13:186–188.

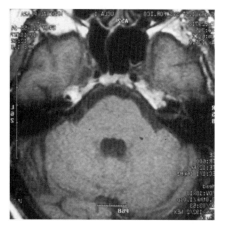

FIGURE 83.1A

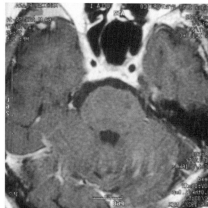

FIGURE 83.1B

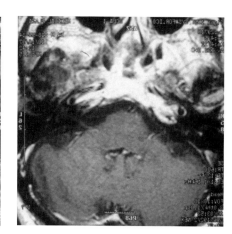

FIGURE 83.1C

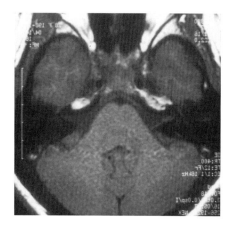

FIGURE 83.2A

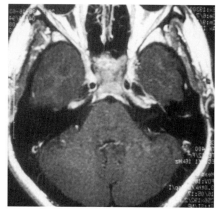

FIGURE 83.2B

CLINICAL HISTORY

A 37-year-old man presents with acute onset of left-sided facial nerve palsy and ipsilateral otalgia. Otoscopic examination discloses a vesicular eruption in the external auditory canal.

FINDINGS

Contrast-enhanced T1-weighted axial images through the temporal bone show thickening and enhancement in the porus acusticus (Fig. 83.1A), the geniculate ganglion (Fig. 83.1B), and the mastoid segment of the left facial nerve (Fig. 83.1C). No abnormal enhancement is seen in the right facial nerve.

Axial precontrast (Fig. 83.2A) and postcontrast (Fig. 83.2B) T1-weighted images show faint linear enhancement in the tympanic segment of the left facial nerve in a patient with no symptoms related to the facial nerve.

DIAGNOSIS

Ramsay-Hunt syndrome (herpes zoster otticus).

DISCUSSION

Herpes zoster otticus is a herpetic inflammation of the geniculate ganglion described by J. Ramsay-Hunt in 1907. After it was recognized that other cranial nerves (V, VIII, and X) could also be affected, a more general term "herpes zoster cephalicus" arose as did an array of confusing terminology designating several subgroups of the disease.

This viral induced neuronitis is thought to result from reactivation of herpes zoster viruses lodged in the geniculate ganglion in a dormant state, usually triggered by a nonspecific event such as stress, a transient immunodeficiency, or superinfection with a heterotopic virus. Several factors contribute to the resulting neuronitis. The most favored are a direct immunologic attack leading to a demyelinating neuropathy and a vasculitis of the vasa nervorum causing an ischemic axonal neuropathy. The end result of edema and inflammation is compression of the nerve against the rigid bony walls of the fallopian canal and further aggravation of the ischemic damage.

Clinically, the disease manifests with acute onset of complete facial nerve palsy, usually to a graver degree than the one associated with Bell's palsy. Loss of the special functions of the facial nerve result in loss of lacrimation, hyperacusis, and loss of taste in the anterior two thirds of the tongue. Involvement of cranial nerves V and VIII is not uncommon and may result in facial numbness, sensorineural hearing loss, and vertigo. Serologic testing may disclose an increase in viral antibody titers both in the serum and cerebrospinal fluid, and electromyography and electroneurography may be useful to monitor treatment and to establish the prognosis.

The main role of imaging is to exclude neoplasms in the setting of patients with seventh and eighth nerve symptoms. Imaging findings are nonspecific and, up to this date, have no clear implications in patient management or prognosis. MRI is the only imaging modality able to show inflammatory changes along cranial nerves manifesting by abnormal contrast enhancement.

Differential diagnosis includes, besides herpes zoster otticus, Bell's palsy, infection with human immunodeficiency virus, Lyme disease, syphilis, and sarcoid. Another important differential consideration is perineural spread of tumor. Contrast enhancement along the facial nerve, usually in the tympanic and less commonly in the mastoid segments, is a frequent finding and is due to the presence of a rich circumneural vascular plexus (Fig. 83.2). However, enhancement along the meatal and labyrinthine segments of the facial nerve and in the geniculate ganglion is not seen in normal individuals and proved to be negative prognostic factors in patients with facial nerve palsy.

Hyperemia and damage to the blood–nerve barrier have been postulated as the major causes of facial nerve enhancement in inflammatory neuronitis. Paradoxically, enhancement may be absent at the onset of the disease, probably resulting from ischemia of the vasa nervorum compromising the vascular delivery of the contrast agent. As opposed to neoplasms, the enhancement seen in inflammatory conditions is linear and usually continuous. In Ramsay-Hunt syndrome, enhancement may also be demonstrated within the membranous labyrinth, along the course of the trigeminal nerve, and in the external auditory canal and auricle.

Herpes zoster otticus is treated with a combination of steroids and acyclovir for a period of 10 days and, in most patients, symptoms resolve without sequelae. Surgical decompression of the facial nerve has limited applications, mostly when the diagnosis is in doubt or when symptoms persist or recur in a 6-month period.

SUGGESTED READINGS

Adour KK. Otological complications of herpes zoster. *Ann Neurol* 1994;35(Suppl):S62–S64.

Ramsey KL, Kasef LG. Role of magnetic resonance imaging in the diagnosis of bilateral facial nerve palsy. *Am J Otol* 1993;14:605–609.

Tada Y, Aoyagi M, Tojima H, et al. Gd-DTPA enhanced MRI in Ramsay-Hunt syndrome. *Acta Otolaryngol Suppl* 1994;511:170–174.

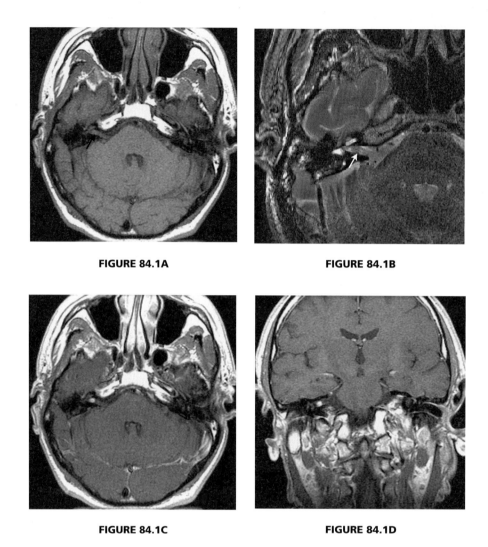

FIGURE 84.1A

FIGURE 84.1B

FIGURE 84.1C

FIGURE 84.1D

CLINICAL HISTORY

A 51-year-old man presents with sensorineural hearing loss.

FINDINGS

T1-weighted MRI shows a small soft tissue mass in the right internal auditory canal (IAC) (Fig. 84.1A). The T2-weighted image shows a filling defect in the normal cerebrospinal fluid (CSF) signal at that location (Fig. 84.1B). Following gadolinium administration, there is focal enhancement of the mass (Fig. 84.1C, D).

DIAGNOSIS

Intracanalicular vestibular schwannoma.

DISCUSSION

This lesion has been described by a variety of names, most commonly "acoustic neuroma." This name is inaccurate in that most of the lesions are neither neuromas nor do they arise from the acoustic nerve. The preferred term is *vestibular schwannoma.*

A schwannoma is a benign neoplasm of the nerve sheath. It is encapsulated and composed of Schwann cells. A neurofibroma is also a benign neoplasm; however, it is unencapsulated and is composed of both Schwann cells and proliferating axons. There are also other microscopic features that generally allow these lesions to be distinguished.

Vestibular schwannomas arise from the Schwann cells of (most often) the vestibular branch of the eighth cranial nerve, usually within the IAC (at the glial-schwann cell junction). They account for 5% to 10% of all intracranial tumors and 80% to 90% of tumors in the cerebellopontine angle. The eighth nerve is the most common cranial nerve to give rise to schwannomas. Intracanalicular schwannomas comprise approximately 10% of all vestibular schwannomas at imaging diagnosis.

Patients present most frequently in the fifth to sixth decade, with males and females being equally affected. Because these are slow-growing tumors, clinical symptoms can have a gradual onset and many patients have had otologic symptoms for years before seeking medical attention. The most common presenting symptoms are unilateral sensorineural hearing loss, tinnitus, and unsteady gait. Less frequently, there are signs of cranial nerve compression and increased intracranial pressure.

Larger tumors with significant growth into the CPA can be visualized by either contrast-enhanced CT or MRI. MRI, however, is the study of choice for evaluating suspected intracanalicular tumors. On axial T2-weighted images, the normal eighth cranial nerve is seen within the IAC as a linear structure of signal intensity similar to that of the brain.

Small intracanalicular schwannomas can be seen best on T1-weighted images with higher signal intensity than normal nerve and surrounding CSF or as a filling defect on high resolution T2-weighted image. MRI with gadolinium is an effective method for evaluating these lesions.

Although vestibular schwannomas are the most common neoplasm in the IAC, other possibilities should be considered in a patient with an intracanalicular lesion. Some patients with clinical and radiologic findings indicative of an intracanalicular schwannoma have been found to have nonneoplastic inflammation of the nerve at surgery. Some of these lesions either are not progressive or resolve spontaneously. For this reason, and because most acoustic tumors tend to grow slowly, many experts advocate follow-up MRI at 6 to 12 months in patients with intracanalicular lesions with stable clinical symptoms before any surgical intervention is instituted.

Other lesions should also be considered, especially if the patient presents with symptoms other than deafness or tinnitus. Neuromas of other cranial nerves, meningiomas, cholesteatomas, metastatic tumors, lipomas, and other vascular lesions can also occupy this space.

The preferred treatment for vestibular schwannoma is surgical excision. The most common complications of surgery include hearing loss and facial nerve damage. Stereotactic radiosurgery is a noninvasive approach used in some patients to arrest the growth. Preliminary studies show complication rates similar to those seen with surgery.

SUGGESTED READINGS

Han ME, Lufkin R, Jabour B, et al. Non-neoplastic enhancing lesions mimicking intracanalicular acoustic neuroma on Gd enhanced MR. *Radiology* 1991;179:795–796.

Rowland LP, et al. *Merritt's textbook of neurology,* 8th ed. Philadelphia: Lea & Febiger, 1989;288–290.

Sidman JD, et al. Gadolinium. The new gold standard for diagnosing cerebellopontine angle tumors. *Arch Otolaryngol Head Neck Surg* 1989;115:1244–1247.

Valvassori GE. Diagnosis of retrocochlear and central vestibular disease by magnetic resonance imaging. *Ann Otol Rhinol Laryngol* 1988;97:19–22.

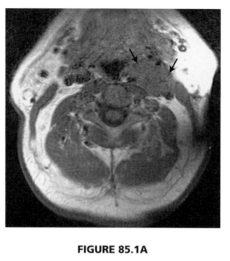

FIGURE 85.1A

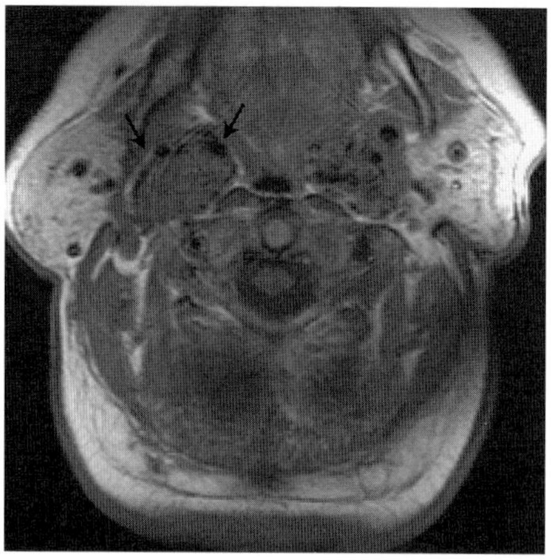

FIGURE 85.1B

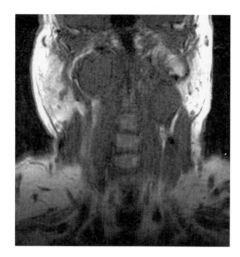

FIGURE 85.1C

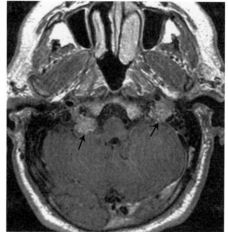

FIGURE 85.1D

CLINICAL HISTORY

A 56-year-old man presents with lower cranial nerve paralysis in the right side.

FINDINGS

The axial T1-weighted image shows a left-sided mass centered in the bifurcation of the carotid arteries (Fig. 85.1A). A scan slightly higher shows a second right-sided mass displacing these vessels anteriorly (Fig. 85.1B). Their relative positions are visible on the coronal view (Fig. 85.1C). A higher axial view postcontrast through the jugular foramen shows bilateral enhancing masses (Fig. 85.1D).

DIAGNOSIS

Left carotid body tumor, right glomus vagale, and bilateral glomus jugulare tumors.

DISCUSSION

A paraganglioma is a slowly growing neuroendocrine endoplasm that arises from neural crest derivatives. *Chemodectoma, glomus tumor, nonchromaffin paraganglioma,* and *neurocristopathic tumor* are the most common names given to this lesion. The precapillary arteriovenous shunts and nonchromaffin cells are characteristic of the histologic appearance of these tumors.

Paragangliomas can be classified by their locations: tympanic, jugular, carotid, and vagal. There is a tendency of multicentricity of tumors (10%), especially in a patient with a carotid body showing familial tendency (26%). The incidence of true malignancy showing metastasis is higher in a carotid body tumor (10%) than the overall incidence, which varies from 2% to 6%. The biologic behavior or natural course of the tumors is not clearly correlated with histologic appearances.

The clinical findings of paragangliomas are slowly growing and compressible masses or cranial nerve paralysis, according to the location. In a temporal lesion, conductive or sensorineural hearing loss or pulsatile tinnitus may be the initial symptom, and a vertically fixed and laterally movable mass is a characteristic finding in a carotid body tumor.

Radiologic diagnosis of this tumor is based on the location of tumor and characteristic hypervascularity. For the evaluation of temporal bone, thin-slice, high-resolution CT is the imaging modality of choice; however, in other locations, MRI has some advantages in delineating and characterizing the lesion with its superb soft tissue contrast. The hypervascular nature of the tumor can be demonstrated by MRI with signal void of flowing vessel.

Surgery is the therapy of choice for most patients with single lesions. Even though conventional angiography is generally no longer used for diagnosis, preoperative embolization is used in most cases to limit bleeding at surgery. Radiation therapy is used in some patients who are not surgical candidates. (See also specific case discussions on carotid body tumors, glomus jugulare, and glomus vagale.)

SUGGESTED READINGS

Bastounis E, Maltezos C, Pikoulis E, et al. Surgical treatment of carotid body tumours. *Eur J Surg* 1999;165:198–202.

Larson TC II, Reese DF, Baker HL Jr, et al. Glomus tympanicum chemodectomas: radiographic and clinical characteristics. *Radiology* 1987;163:801–806.

Netterville JL, Reilly KM, Robertson D, et al. Carotid body tumors: a review of 30 patients with 46 tumors. *Laryngoscope* 1995;105:115–126.

Olsen WL, Dillon WP, Kelly WM, et al. MR imaging of paragangliomas. *AJNR Am J Neuroradiol* 1986;7:1039–1042.

Rodraiguez-Cuevas S, Laopez-Garza J, Labastida-Almendaro S. Carotid body tumors in inhabitants of altitudes higher than 2000 meters above sea level. *Head Neck* 1998;20:374–378.

Shugar MA, Mafee MF. Diagnosis of carotid body tumors in dynamic computerized tomography. *Head Neck Surg* 1982;4:518–521.

Som PM, Sacher M, Stollman AL, et al. Common tumor of the parapharyngeal space: refined imaging diagnosis. *Radiology* 1988;169:81–85.

Vogl T, Bruning R, Schedel H, et al. Paragangliomas of the jugular bulb and carotid body: MR imaging with short sequences and GD-DTPA enhancement. *AJNR Am J Neuroradiol* 1989;10:823–827.

Win T, Lewin JS. Imaging characteristics of carotid body tumors. *Am J Otolaryngol* 1995;16:325–328.

Zak FG, Lawson W. *The paraganglionic chemoreceptor system. Physiology, pathology, and clinical medicine.* New York: Springer-Verlag, 1982;267–285.

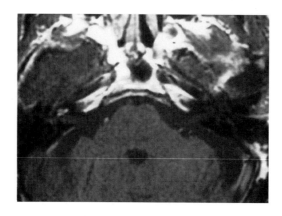

FIGURE 86.1A

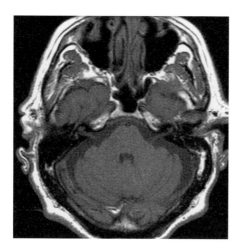

FIGURE 86.1B

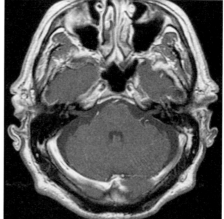

FIGURE 86.1C

CLINICAL HISTORY

A 60-year-old man presents with sensorineural hearing loss on the right. Four months later, symptoms resolve.

FINDINGS

On axial T1-weighted MR postcontrast image, there is focal enhancement of the cochlea. No increased signal was present on the precontrast views (Fig. 86.1A). On the precontrast and postcontrast T1-weighted images obtained 4 months later, these findings are resolved (Fig. 86.1B, C).

DIAGNOSIS

Labyrinthitis.

DISCUSSION

A nonneoplastic lesion may cause contrast enhancement of a cranial nerve or labyrinthine structures on MRI, mimicking, for example, schwannoma. The possible enhancement mechanisms are disruption of the blood–nerve and labyrinthine barrier and hypervascularity or hyperemia of the perineural tissue. Many cases show diffuse enhancement of the nerves along their course, so the radiologic diagnosis of inflammatory lesion may be possible. However, this case shows focal intralabyrinthine enhancement of the cochlea. The fact that the lesion resolved with time helps to confirm its inflammatory nature.

SUGGESTED READINGS

Anderson RE, Laskoff JM. Ramsay Hunt syndrome mimicking intracanalicular acoustic neuroma on contrast-enhanced MR. *AJNR Am J Neuroradiol* 1990;11:409.

Daniels DL, Czervionke LF, Millen SJ, et al. MR imaging of facial nerve enhancement in Bell's palsy or after temporal bone surgery. *Radiology* 1989;171:807–809.

Han ME, Lufkin R, Jabour B, et al. Non-neoplastic enhancing lesions mimicking intracanalicular acoustic neuroma on Gd enhanced MR. *Radiology* 1991;179:795–796.

Tien R, Dillon WP, Jackler RK. Contrast-enhanced MR imaging of the facial nerve in 11 patients with Bell's palsy. *AJNR Am J Neuroradiol* 1990;11:735–741.

Tien R, Dillon WP. Herpes trigeminal neuritis and rhombencephalitis on Gd-DTPA-enhanced MR imaging. *AJNR Am J Neuroradiol* 1990;11:413–414.

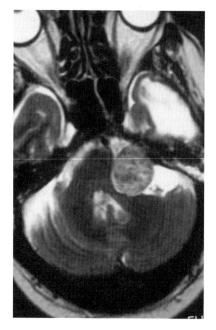

FIGURE 87.1A

FIGURE 87.1B

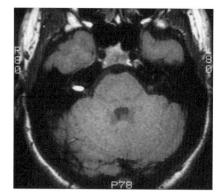

FIGURE 87.2

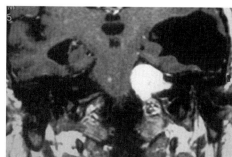

FIGURE 87.1C

CLINICAL HISTORY

A 67-year-old man presents with left-sided hearing loss and tinnitus.

FINDINGS

Axial T2-weighted and axial and coronal postcontrast T1-weighted images through the cerebellopontine angle (Fig. 87.1A–C) show a large, homogeneously enhancing mass in the left cerebellopontine angle cistern centered at the porus acusticus with a small funnel shaped intracanalicular component. The tumor indents the middle cerebellar peduncle and left aspect of the pons and deforms the fourth ventricle. A large posttraumatic porencephalic cavity is incidentally noted in the left temporal lobe.

An axial postgadolinium T1-weighted image of another patient (Fig. 87.2) shows an intensely enhancing tubular lesion in the right internal auditory canal extending from the porus acusticus to the fundus of the internal auditory canal.

DIAGNOSIS

Vestibular schwannoma.

DISCUSSION

Vestibular schwannomas account for 90% of all intracranial schwannomas and for 80% to 90% of all cerebellopontine angle tumors. They are more prevalent between the fourth and seventh decades, have a slight female gender predominance, and have a family history of acoustic tumors in 10% of patients.

Bilateral vestibular schwannomas are diagnostic of neurofibromatosis type II.

The designation "vestibular schwannoma" results from the fact that most tumors arise from the inferior division of the vestibular nerve, usually in the vicinity of the Scarpa's ganglion. They are benign, slow-growing tumors with a reported growth rate ranging from 0.1 to 0.2 cm per year. Vestibular schwannomas may occur anywhere along the course of the nerve from the ventrolateral aspect of the pons to the vestibule. At the time of presentation, most tumors are mixed, having cisternal and intracanalicular components, followed in frequency by purely intracanalicular and purely cisternal tumors. Intralabyrinthine schwannomas, usually located in the vestibule, may also occur but are much less common.

Symptoms result from compression of nerve fibers and compromise of vascular supply. High-frequency sensorineural hearing loss is frequently the presenting sign, followed by vertigo and tinnitus. Large tumors compressing the basilar cisterns, brainstem, fourth ventricle, and cerebellum may present with disequilibrium, ataxia, headaches, and other cranial nerve deficits, usually from the seventh and fifth nerves. Intratumoral hemorrhage leading to acute mass effect is responsible for sudden hearing loss and occurs in 10% of cases.

MRI is currently the "gold standard" for the diagnosis of acoustic tumors, sometimes detecting tumors as small as 1 to 2 mm in size. Although several highly T2-weighted MR sequences (tridimensional Fourier transform [3DFT] and construction interference in the steady state [CISS]) have proved to be very sensitive in the detection of small tumors as small filling defects within the fluid-filled internal auditory canal, contrast-enhanced T1-weighted images remain the MR gold standard for small tumor detection. Most vestibular schwannomas present as ice cream cone–shaped lesions, with the "cone" representing the intracanalicular component and the "ice cream" being the cisternal component. Large tumors are usually heterogeneous in signal with areas of cystic degeneration and, sometimes, hemorrhage. Purely intracanalicular tumors are homogeneous, cylindrical in shape, and vividly enhancing. When small, they may be difficult to differentiate from inflammatory conditions. Remodeling or enlargement of the internal auditory canal and the presence of a convex medial border favors the diagnosis of tumor.

CT is useful in a presurgical setting to provide the surgeon with bony anatomic landmarks. Large tumors usually lead to flaring or erosion of the internal auditory canal, which is best seen on CT.

Major differential considerations for cerebellopontine angle lesions include meningiomas, other cranial nerve schwannomas, and epidermoid cysts. The presence of a large dural based tumor, eccentric relative to the internal auditory canal and forming obtuse angles with the temporal bone, favors the diagnosis of a cerebellopontine angle meningioma.

Management of vestibular schwannomas depends on the size, location, and degree of serviceable hearing. Surgery remains the treatment of choice, although radiosurgery is being increasingly used with a high rate of tumor control. Conservative management is also a possibility, particularly in older patients if an adequate follow-up is guaranteed.

SUGGESTED READINGS

Casselman JW, Kuhweide R, Dehaene I, et al. Magnetic resonance examination of the inner ear and cerebellopontine angle in patients with vertigo and/or abnormal findings at vestibular testing. *Acta Radiol Suppl* 1994;513:15–27.

Guirado CR, Martinez P, Roig R, et al. Three dimensional MR of the inner ear with steady state free precession. *AJNR Am J Neuroradiol* 1995;16:1909–1913.

Mafee MF. MR imaging of intralabyrinthine schwannoma, labyrinthites and other labyrinthine pathology. *Otolaryngol Clin North Am* 1995;28:407–430.

Mark AS, Fitzgerald D. MR of the inner ear. *Baillieres Clin Neurol* 1994;3:515–535.

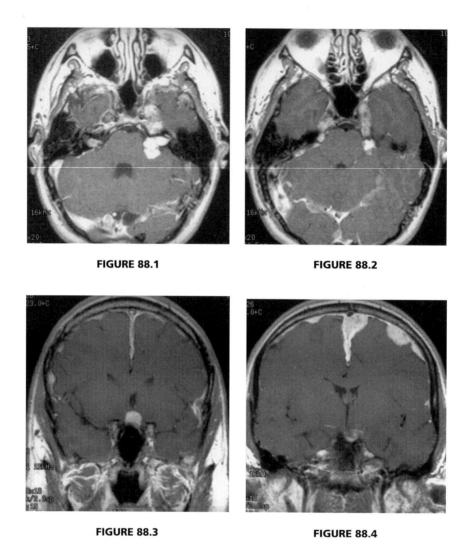

FIGURE 88.1

FIGURE 88.2

FIGURE 88.3

FIGURE 88.4

CLINICAL HISTORY

A 36-year-old woman presents with progressive visual loss. She also has a history of pseudotumor cerebri.

FINDINGS

Contrast-enhanced images show enhancing masses in the internal auditory canal and cavernous sinuses bilaterally (Fig. 88.1). The enhancing mass in the left cavernous sinus extends to the prepontine cistern along the trigeminal nerve (Fig. 88.2). In addition, a well-defined homogeneously enhancing mass is evident at the tuberculum sella (Fig. 88.3). Numerous diffuse dural based lesions are present along the falx and over the cerebral convexities bilaterally (Fig. 88.4).

DIAGNOSIS

Neurofibromatosis type II (NFII).

DISCUSSION

NFII is an autosomal dominant disease transmitted on chromosome 22. It is much less common than NF type I (NFI) and occurs in approximately 1 in 50,000 live births. Bilateral acoustic neuromas are hallmarks of this disease. Diagnosis is made when the patient has either (a) bilateral acoustic neuromas or (b) first degree relative with NFII and either a single acoustic neuroma or any of two of the following: schwannomas, neurofibromas, meningiomas, or ependymomas. Next to cranial nerve VIII, the cranial nerve V is the second most common site of schwannoma. Spine lesions in NFII are fairly common. Intramedullary spinal lesion is usually ependymoma. Intradural extramedullary lesions are either meningioma or schwannoma in NFII. Other radiographic findings include dural ectasia of the internal auditory canal or spine (lateral thoracic meningocele) and prominent calcification of the choroid plexus. The cutaneous manifestation in NFII is much less common than in NFI; therefore, diagnosis is usually made later in life.

In this case, superior sagittal sinus thrombosis developed secondary to meningioma, resulting in poor venous drainage and subsequent pseudotumor cerebri. (See Case 80 for a more detailed discussion of NFII.)

SUGGESTED READINGS

Elster AD. Radiologic screening in neurocutaneous syndrome: strategies and controversies. *AJNR Am J Neuroradiol* 1992;13:1078–1082.

National Institute of Health Consensus Development Conference. Neurofibromatosis conference statement. *Arch Neurol* 1988;45:579–588.

Smirniotopoulos JG, Murphy FM. The phakomatoses. *AJNR Am J Neuroradiol* 1992;13:725–746.

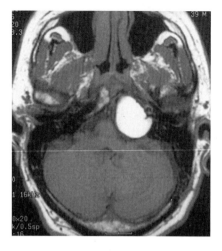

FIGURE 89.1

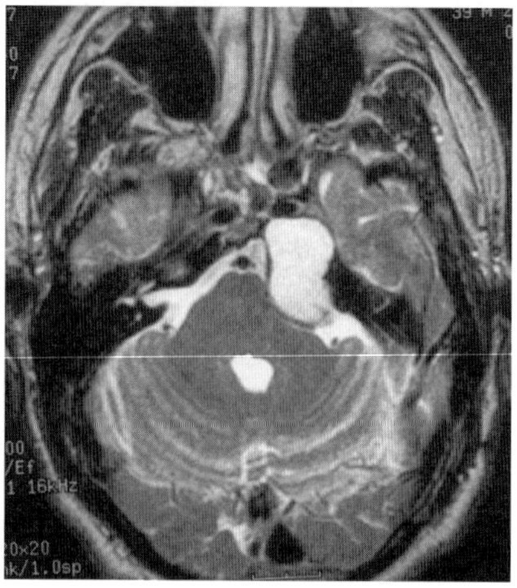

FIGURE 89.2

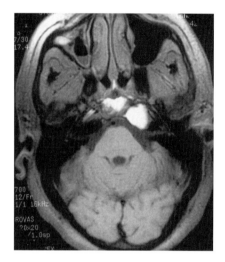

FIGURE 89.3

FIGURE 89.4

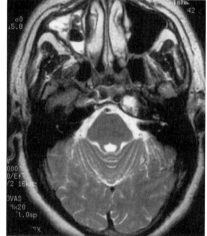

CLINICAL HISTORY

A 39-year-old man presents with left lateral gaze diplopia.

FINDINGS

Noncontrast T1-weighted image shows a well-defined mass high in T1 signal at the left petrous apex. Mild mass effect is seen upon the left lateral pontomedullary junction without edema (Fig. 89.1). The lesion is also markedly hyperintense on T2-weighted images with dark signal rim at the posterior border (Fig. 89.2). No pathologic contrast enhancement is seen (postcontrast image not shown).

DIAGNOSIS

Cholesterol granuloma (cholesterol cyst).

DISCUSSION

A cholesterol granuloma typically arises from the petrous apex of the temporal bone. The cholesterol granuloma is a clinical entity entirely distinct from cholesteatoma. The pathogenesis of a cholesterol granuloma is believed to be due to repeated hemorrhage after acute or subacute middle ear infection, associated with foreign body reaction.

On histopathologic examination, a granulomatous reaction to blood debris is present, including cholesterol clefts, hemosiderin, foreign body cells, pigment-collecting macrophages, and foam cells (lipid-laden macrophages) surrounded by a fibrous connective tissue (acquired cholesteatoma is encapsulated by squamous epithelium). Three factors are considered to play an important role in its development: (a) hemorrhage, (b) interference with drainage, and (c) obstruction of ventilation of the middle ear.

Following a course of acute or subacute otomastoiditis and resultant accumulation of mucosal secretion, there may be hemorrhage resulting from congestion of the vessels (hyperemia). The blood-breakdown byproducts are then the main source of cholesterol and initiate a foreign body reaction. Recurrent bleeding from these vessels or necrosis of local tissue continues the cycle, enlarging the lesions.

CT and MRI have made it possible to make a strong presumptive diagnosis of cholesterol granuloma and congenital cholesteatoma (epidermoid) of the petrous apex. The cholesterol granuloma appears markedly bright on T1- and T2-weighted images because of hemorrhagic product with occasional T2 low signal rim of hemosiderin deposition. Cholesterol granuloma is a well-defined expansile lesion in the petrous apex with bone remodeling on CT.

The differential diagnosis includes mucocele of the petrous apex and petrous apicitis, because signal characteristics of mucocele or inflammatory disease depend on degree of hydration and proteinaceous material content.

SUGGESTED READINGS

Friedman I. Epidermoid cholesteatoma and cholesterol granuloma: experimental and human. *Ann Otol Rhinol Laryngol* 1959;68:57–79.

Lo WW, et al. CT diagnosis of cholesterol granuloma of the petrous apex, with discussion of pathological and surgical considerations. *Radiology* 1984;153:705–711.

Shikhani AH, et al. Pathologic quiz case 2. Cholesterol granuloma of the temporal bone. *Arch Otolaryngol Head Neck Surg* 1989;115:1476–1478.

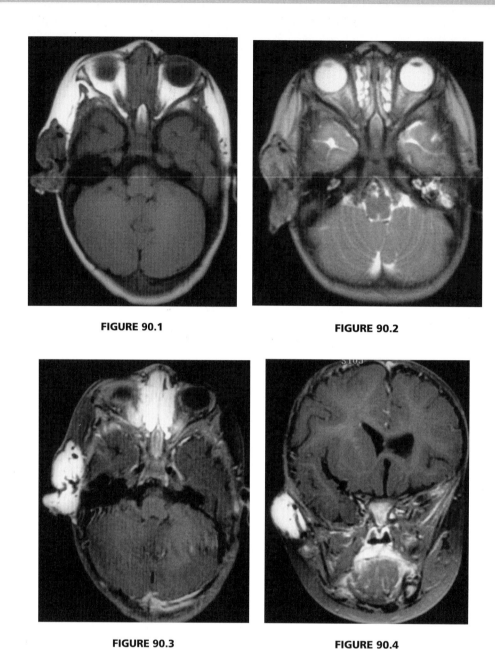

FIGURE 90.1

FIGURE 90.2

FIGURE 90.3

FIGURE 90.4

CLINICAL HISTORY

A 10-month-old girl has an enlarging mass over the right pinna.

FINDINGS

T1- and T2-weighted images demonstrate an exophilic mass over the right earlobe that has low signal on T1-weighted images and slightly high signal on T2-weighted images (Figs. 90.1, 90.2). There are serpentine areas of flow voids in the medial aspect of the mass, consistent with presence of arterial feeding vessels. However, the superficial portion of the mass appears more solid without flow voids, associated with marked contrast enhancement (Figs. 90.3, 90.4).

DIAGNOSIS

Presumed infantile hemangioma (capillary hemangioma).

DISCUSSION

Capillary hemangiomas are benign vascular endothelial tumors that primarily occur in infants, with a significant female predominance (5:1). They typically grow during the first year of life and usually regress thereafter, before the child is 5 years old.

MRI is the examination of choice for hemangioma, because the lesion appears as markedly hyperintense on T2-weighted image, associated with intense contrast enhancement. Capillary hemangiomas may have many small arterial supplies containing flow voids on MRI. Rarely, capillary hemangiomas cause arterial hemorrhage. Patients should be observed until the lesion regresses. Angiogram is not performed until treatment is necessary. This patient has been clinically followed up without intervention.

Cavernous hemangioma, on the other hand, is commonly seen in adults (second to fourth decades of life) and slowly progresses. Cavernous hemangiomas are composed of large dilated vascular channels surrounded by thin endothelial cells. Cavernous hemangioma appears as a well-defined but sometimes infiltrative mass on MRI. The prominent arterial supply seen in capillary hemangiomas is absent. These lesions show intense enhancement with contrast. T2-weighted image typically shows a distinctive high signal striated or septated configuration. This correlates with interspersed fibrous and fatty septa between the vascular channels. A pathognomonic finding on CT is presence of phleboliths; however, these are more difficult to recognize on MRI.

SUGGESTED READINGS

Herbreteau D, Aymard A, Jhaveri HS, et al. Current management of cervicofacial superficial vascular malformations and hemangiomas. In Connors JJ, Wojak JC, eds. *Interventional neuroradiology: strategies and practical techniques.* Philadelphia: WB Saunders, 1999;317–337.

Mafee MF, Putterman A, Valvassori GE, et al. Orbital space-occupying lesions: role of CT and MRI. Analysis of 145 cases. *Radiol Clin North Am* 1987;24:529–559.

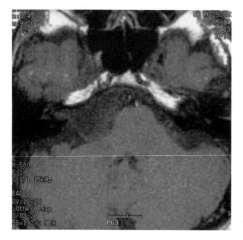

FIGURE 91.1

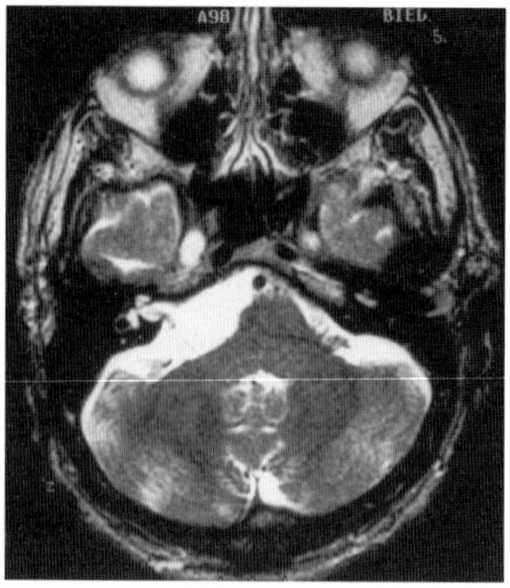

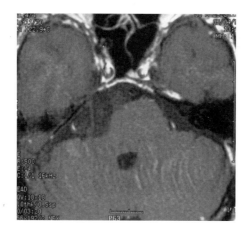

FIGURE 91.2

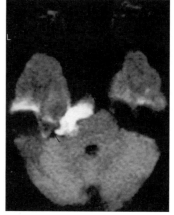

FIGURE 91.3

FIGURE 91.4

CLINICAL HISTORY

A 56-year-old man presents with right trigeminal nerve paresthesia.

FINDINGS

There is a well-defined hypointense mass in the right cerebellopontine angle compressing the lateral aspect of the pons (Figs. 91.1, 91.2). The lesion is isointense to cerebrospinal fluid (CSF) on T2-weighted image, but slightly hyperintense to CSF on T1-weighted image. No contrast enhancement is seen. Note that the right trigeminal nerve is stretched and displaced laterally by the mass (Fig. 91.3). Diffusion weighted image shows marked hyperintense lesion, indicating that the lesion has restricted diffusion (Fig. 91.4).

DIAGNOSIS

Epidermoid.

DISCUSSION

Epidermoids (developmental cholesteatomas) are derived from incomplete separation of the neural and cutaneous ectoderm at the time of closure of the neural tube. The bulk of the tumor is composed of desquamated cellular debris, consisting of keratin, lipids, and cholesterol. The capsule of epidermoid is lined by a single layer of squamous epithelium. The common sites are the cerebellopontine angle cistern (40%), the suprasellar cistern, and the pineal region.

Epidermoids account for 5% of cerebellopontine angle tumors. They are slow-growing benign lesions that expand gradually. A patient with epidermoid usually presents with cranial nerve dysfunction, such as facial pain, facial palsy, diplopia, and hearing loss. Epidermoids may encase the neurovascular structures through the cerebellopontine angle, rather than displace them. Extradural epidermoids are much less common than intradural epidermoids. These occur in the temporal bone, petrous apex, and diploic space of the calvarium.

T1-weighted image reveals a well-defined mass with signal intensity intermediate between brain and CSF, with no contrast enhancement. On T2-weighted image, the lesion appears nearly isointense to CSF; however, heterogeneity in the lesion can be seen. Diffusion weighted imaging and fluid-attenuated inversion recovery (FLAIR) imaging sequences show that epidermoids do not follow CSF in signal intensity and therefore are useful in differentiating epidermoid from arachnoid cyst.

Differential diagnoses include arachnoid cyst, cystic acoustic neuroma, dermoid (usually fatty signal characteristics), and neuroenteric cyst. Lack of contrast enhancement and high signal on diffusion weighted and FLAIR sequence are keys for radiologic diagnosis.

SUGGESTED READINGS

Gao P, Obborn AG, Smirniotopulos JG, et al. Radiologic-pathologic correlation: epidermoid tumor of the cerebellopontine angle. *AJNR Am J Neuroradiol* 1992;13:863–872.

Mohanty A, Verkatrama SK, Rao BR, et al. Experience with cerebellopontine angle epidermoids. *Neurosurgery* 1997;40:24–30.

Sakamoto Y, Takahashi M, Ushio Y, et al. Visibility of epidermoid tumors on steady state free precession images. *AJNR Am J Neuroradiol* 1994;15:1737–1744.

Tampieri D, Melanson D, Ethier R. MR imaging of epidermoid cysts. *AJNR Am J Neuroradiol* 1989;10:352–356.

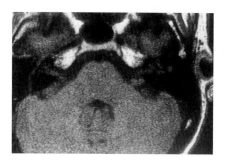

FIGURE 92.1A

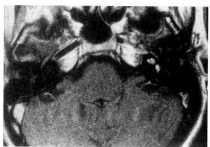

FIGURE 92.1B

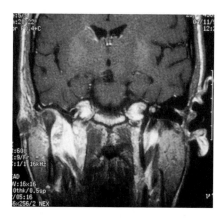

FIGURE 92.1C

CLINICAL HISTORY

A 35-year-old man presents with acute onset of vertigo, nausea, and vomiting. An audiogram discloses severe left-sided sensorineural hearing loss.

FINDINGS

Axial T1-weighted (Fig. 92.1A) and axial and coronal gadolinium-enhanced images (Fig. 92.1B, C) through the temporal bone show intense linear enhancement in the membranous labyrinth involving the basal and apical turns of the cochlea and the vestibule. There is no abnormal enhancement in the semicircular canals or within the internal auditory canal, and there is no abnormal meningeal enhancement. The middle ear cavity and mastoid air cells are clear. The right membranous labyrinth is normal and shows no enhancement.

DIAGNOSIS

Labyrinthitis.

DISCUSSION

Labyrinthitis is defined as an inflammatory process of the membranous labyrinth which may have several etiologies. The viral etiology is the most common, followed by bacterial, syphilitic, and granulomatous infections. Some forms of the disease in which no infectious agent is found (idiopathic forms) have recently been attributed to an autoimmune process.

The diagnosis in this situation is made by a positive lymphocyte transformation test and a positive response to steroids. Because of its location between the intracranial compartment and the tympanic cavity, the labyrinth may be affected by infectious processes arising from the meninges (meningogenic labyrinthitis), middle ear cavity (tympanogenic labyrinthitis), or through a hematogenic route. Labyrinthitis may also be iatrogenic, usually after surgery or trauma. Cerebrospinal fluid spread of meningitic infections may occur via internal auditory canal, which communicates with the endolymph within the vestibule or via cochlear aqueduct, which communicates with the perilymph within the scala tympani at the basal turn of the cochlea.

Tympanogenic infections (otitis media) may spread to the membranous labyrinth through the oval and round windows or, in the presence of aggressive cholesteatomas, through labyrinthine fistulas to the lateral semicircular canal. Hematogenous dissemination is uncommon and is usually associated with measles and mumps. Whereas most meningogenic and hematogenic labyrinthitis tend to be bilateral, tympanogenic processes are usually unilateral.

Patients present clinically with acute onset of vertigo and sensorineural hearing loss. A thorough clinical history and the presence of other symptoms and signs may point to the cause and mechanism of the disease.

Differential diagnosis includes labyrinthine fistulas (iatrogenic, traumatic, or resulting from a cholesteatoma), ischemic events affecting the labyrinth, primary tumors (such as intralabyrinthine schwannomas), and secondary invasion of the labyrinth through direct spread of adjacent tumors (such as paragangliomas and adenocarcinomas of the endolymphatic sac). Metastases to the labyrinth may also occur.

In the acute phase, MR findings include diffuse or focal linear enhancement within the membranous labyrinth, involving the vestibule or cochlea and correlating with clinical findings. Labyrinthine enhancement is always pathologic and is never seen in normal individuals. MR studies should always include precontrast T1- and T2-weighted images to exclude intralabyrinthine hemorrhage, particularly in the setting of trauma, coagulopathy, or neoplasm.

Labyrinthine fistula on MRI may manifest as an area of focal enhancement at the fistulous site and, in this situation, CT is useful to detect pneumolabyrinth and effusions within the middle ear cavity. Associated enhancement of the seventh and eighth nerves suggests herpes zoster otticus or Ramsay-Hunt syndrome. Intravestibular schwannomas usually manifest as a focal nodular area of enhancement.

Management depends on the mechanism of injury, and therapy should be aimed to the etiologic agent. Although some processes are self-limited and may recover spontaneously with supportive therapy, adequate treatment is still needed to prevent chronicity with a resulting "dead ear." Steroids and steroids combined with antiviral agents have been recommended for autoimmune and viral causes, respectively.

SUGGESTED READINGS

Casselman JW, Kuhweide R, Dehaene I, et al. Magnetic resonance examination of the inner ear and cerebellopontine angle in patients with vertigo and/or abnormal findings at vestibular testing. *Acta Otolaryngol Suppl* 1994;513:15–27.

Maffee MF. MR imaging of intralabyrinthine schwannoma, labyrinthitis and other labyrinthine pathology. *Otolaryngol Clin North Am* 1995;28:407–430.

Marc AS, Fitzgerald D. MRI of the inner ear. *Baillieres Clin Neurol* 1994;3:515–535.

Marc AS, Fitzgerald D. Segmental enhancement of the cochlea on contrast-enhanced MR: correlation with the frequency of hearing loss and possible sign of perilymphatic fistula and autoimmune labyrinthitis. *AJNR Am J Neuroradiol* 1993;14:991–996.

Wilson DE, Talbot JM, Hodgson RS. Magnetic resonance imaging-enhancing lesions of the labyrinth and facial nerve. Clinical correlation. *Arch Otolaryngol Head Neck Surg* 1994;120:560–564.

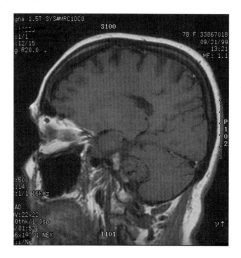

FIGURE 93.1

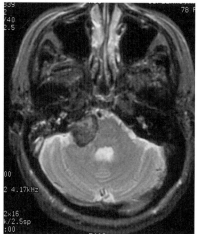

FIGURE 93.2

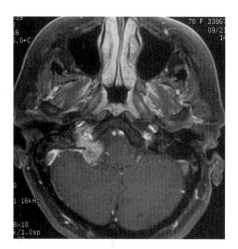

FIGURE 93.3

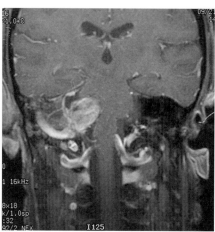

FIGURE 93.4

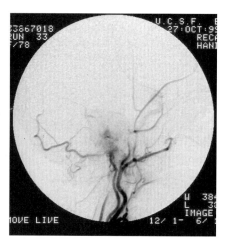

FIGURE 93.5

CLINICAL HISTORY

A 77-year-old woman presents with right-sided deafness for several years.

FINDINGS

Sagittal T1-weighted (Fig. 93.1) and axial T2-weighted (Fig. 93.2) images reveal a mass in the right jugular fossa with significant intracranial extension into the right cerebellopontine angle and compression of the brainstem and cerebellum. The mass has foci of high and low signal intensity in a so-called salt and pepper pattern, and they demonstrate intense contrast enhancement (Figs. 93.3, 93.4). The right mastoid air cells are partially opacified. Selective angiography of the right external carotid artery shows a hypervascular tumor with arterial supply primarily from the ascending pharyngeal and occipital branches (Fig. 93.5).

DIAGNOSIS

Glomus jugulare tumor.

DISCUSSION

Glomus tumors, also commonly known as *chemodectomas* and *nonchromaffin paragangliomas,* are slowly growing neuroendocrine neoplasms, arising from the nonchromaffin paraganglia cells of neural crest derivatives. Glomus tumors are classified by their locations. In the case of glomus jugulare, the tumors may arise from within or adjacent to the jugular vein or from glomus bodies paralleling the tympanic branch of the glossopharyngeal nerve and the auricular branch of the vagus nerve (the nerves of Jacobson and Arnold).

Glomus jugulare is the most common tumor in the region of the jugular fossa, and it commonly demonstrates intracranial extension. Because most lesions are benign and slow-growing, they often enlarge and remodel the jugular foramen, growing along the paths of least resistance, burrowing into fissures, grooves, and natural foramina. When large enough, the tumors erode the jugular spine and the caroticojugular crest, and may grow out through the jugular plate into the middle ear cavity, along the inferior tympanic canaliculus and mastoid region, and is thus termed *glomus jugulotympanicum.*

Most patients with glomus jugulare tumors present with otologic symptoms of conductive hearing loss or pulsatile tinnitus. A retrotympanic mass may be seen on clinical examination. Cranial nerve palsies with jugular foramen (Vernet's) syndrome consisting of glossopharyngeal, vagus, or spinal accessory deficits may be present in a minority of patients. As the tumor enlarges, the hypoglossal nerve may also be compromised in the region of the hypoglossal canal (Collet-Sicard's syndrome). Similarly, the facial nerve may also be affected in its mastoid or tympanic segments. In some cases, the tumors may be secreting and patients present with neuroendocrinologic symptoms.

Precapillary arteriovenous shunting and nonchromaffin cells are specific features of these tumors histologically. The cells are well differentiated and arranged in nests (Zellballen) or cords separated by fibrovascular septa. Mitotic figures and substantial pleomorphism may be seen.

CT is the best overall modality for demonstrating the bony changes. The permeative pattern of bony destruction is rather characteristic with irregular, poorly defined margins without calcification or sclerosis. The lesions first involve the jugular fossa and break through the hypotympanum into the middle ear. There may be destruction of the cochlea, petrous apex, and otic capsule structures as well as the internal auditory canal and clivus. Lateral extension can involve the facial nerve canal.

Like other paragangliomas, glomus jugulare tumors are intensely enhancing following contrast administration. MRI is better than CT in evaluating the full extent of the tumors and in differentiating the tumors from vascular abnormalities such as a dehiscence of the jugular bulb or an aberrant internal carotid artery. MRI also helps to distinguish between glomus jugulare and glomus tympanicum tumors, each with a different surgical approach.

Most tumors are well defined, nearly isointense to the brain on T1-weighted image, and primarily homogeneously hyperintense on T2-weighted image when less than 1.5 cm in size. As the tumors grow to more than 2 cm, a salt and pepper pattern may be seen, which is best appreciated on T2-weighted imaging. This appearance reflects the increase in stromal elements (salt) and the serpentine vascular voids (pepper).

Conventional angiography is no longer routinely used for diagnosis but is valuable for preoperative embolization, which dramatically reduces the surgical morbidity related to bleeding. Glomus jugulare tumors are hypervascular with persistent homogeneous reticular staining and arteriovenous shunting. Arterial blood supplies are most frequently derived from branches of the external carotid artery, especially the ascending pharyngeal artery but also the internal maxillary artery, the posterior auricular artery via stylomastoid branch, and the meningeal branch of the occipital artery. Larger tumors may have additional blood supply from the caroticotympanic branches of the internal carotid artery.

Most glomus jugulare tumors are managed surgically with preoperative embolization. In 2% to 4% of patients, malignant transformation occurs with metastasis to regional lymph nodes. When surgery is contraindicated, tumor control may be achieved with radiation therapy.

SUGGESTED READINGS

Olsen WL, Dillon WP, Kelly WM, et al. MR imaging of paragangliomas. *AJNR Am J Neuroradiology* 1986;7:1039–1042.
Weber AL, Mckenna NJ. Radiologic evaluation of the jugular foramen, vascular variants, abnormalities and tumors. *Neuroimaging Clin North Am* 1994;4:579–598.

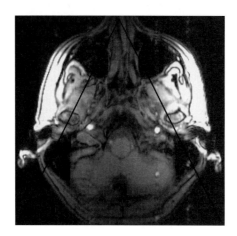

FIGURE 94.1

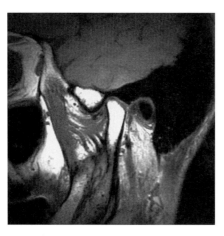

FIGURE 94.2A

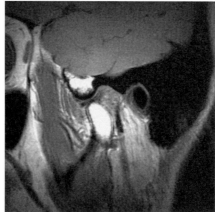

FIGURE 94.2B

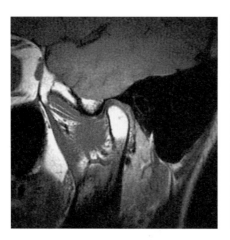

FIGURE 94.3A

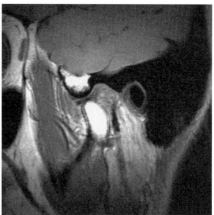

FIGURE 94.3B

CLINICAL HISTORY

A 28-year-old woman presents with pain over the right temporomandibular joint (TMJ) region.

FINDINGS

MRI is performed using oblique sagittal sections with bilateral surface coils in closed and open mouth positions. The axial scout view shows the positions of the oblique sagittal sections (Fig. 94.1). In the right closed mouth position, the disk is in an abnormal position anterior to the condyle (Fig. 94.2A). In the open mouth view, the disk shows persistent anterior displacement (Fig. 94.2B). In comparison, the contralateral side is normal in both the closed and open mouth positions (Fig. 94.3A, B).

DIAGNOSIS

Anterior disk dislocation without reduction.

DISCUSSION

TMJ symptoms are common, with several large series reporting an incidence of up to 30% among adults. A female predominance and a peak incidence of TMJ symptoms in the second decade is consistently reported.

Most cases are idiopathic, although several predisposing factors have been identified. These include dentition problems, arthritides, congenital abnormalities of the condyles, and hyperactivity of the muscles of mastication, such as occurs in bruxism. TMJ derangement is often bilateral because the mandible acts as a single functional unit.

The most frequent symptoms in patients with TMJ derangement are pain, crepitation, and limitation of excursion. Popping during mouth opening, crepitation, pain on palpation of the masticatory muscles, and trismus are obvious on clinical examination.

CT alone using sagittal and coronal reconstructions is not reliable in the diagnosis of disk dislocation because the disk is inconsistently visualized. Conventional or CT arthrography, although accurate in the diagnosis of internal derangement of the TMJ and the only imaging modalities able to reliably diagnose disk perforation or fragmentation, are invasive procedures, with possible complication and patient discomfort. The high resolution and multiplanar capabilities of MRI make it the imaging technique of choice for evaluating internal derangements of the TMJ.

The TMJ is a diarthrodial articulation composed of the mandibular condyle, the glenoid fossa, and the articular eminence of the temporal bone. Between these convex-shaped articular surfaces is a biconcave low signal articular disk. This disk has a "bow tie" morphology with two thick anterior and posterior bands, united by a narrower intermediate zone. The posterior band is connected to the posterior aspect of the articular capsule by fibroelastic tissue containing the neurovascular bundle. This intermediate signal bilaminar zone is responsible for repositioning the disk posteriorly with elevation of the mandible.

A thorough understanding of the normal relationships of the TMJ components is critical in the diagnosis of pathology. In the closed mouth position, the posterior band should be positioned at 12 o'clock relative to the condyle with the intermediate zone between the anterior aspect of the condyle and the articular eminence (Fig. 94.3A). With opening of the mouth, the condyle and disk translate anteriorly and the posterior band lies posterior to the condyle while the intermediate zone is positioned between the tip of the condyle and the articular eminence (Fig. 94.3B).

Internal derangement of the TMJ is a frequent finding and may present a variety of abnormalities in the position and morphology of the disk and articular surfaces. The abnormalities most commonly depicted on imaging studies are anterior dislocation of the disk with or without reduction, combined dislocations (both in the frontal and sagittal planes), acquired and congenital morphologic abnormalities of the condyles, and abnormal excursion of the condyles and disk with opening of the mouth.

The pathophysiologic condition that leads to disk dislocation is increased stretch of the fibroelastic fibers of the bilaminar zone with loss of the ability to exert a restraining force on the disk as the condyle translates forward. The stress exerted on the neurovascular bundle by compression between the condyle and articular eminence leads to pain.

MRI abnormalities should always be correlated with the patient's symptoms and cautiously interpreted; studies demonstrate that roughly 30% of asymptomatic individuals can have abnormalities in disk position and morphology. Imaging findings alone are not diagnostic of disease. Conversely, a normal MRI does not exclude TMJ pathology: internal derangements can be temporarily unstable.

Therapy is aimed at restoring the normal anatomic relationship of the articular elements and maintaining the congruency of the articular surfaces in order to avoid further destruction of articular cartilage. This can be achieved conservatively using splints, anterior repositioning appliances (ARA), and biofeedback techniques. When appropriate, sagittal T1-weighted images with closed and open mouth positions are performed with a corrective splint in place to evaluate the efficacy of the device in reestablishing the normal relationship of the articular elements. Surgery is indicated in cases of protracted chronic dislocations when conservative measures fail to resolve the clinical problem. MRI is the best modality for post-therapeutic follow-up and can evaluate the efficacy of the different therapeutic options.

SUGGESTED READINGS

Brady AP, McDevitt L, Stack JP, et al. A technique for magnetic resonance imaging of the temporomandibular joint. *Clin Radiol* 1993;47:127–133.

Katzberg RW, Westesson PL, Tallents RH, et al. Anatomic disorders of the temporomandibular joint disc in asymptomatic subjects. *J Oral Maxillofac Surg* 1996;54:147–153.

Muller-Leisse C, Augthun M, Bauer W, et al. Anterior disc displacement without reduction in the temporomandibular joint: MRI and associated clinical findings. *J Magn Reson Imaging* 1996;6:769–774.

Rammelsberg P, Pospiech PR, Jager L, et al. Variability of disk position in asymptomatic volunteers and patients with internal derangements of the TMJ. *Oral Surg Oral Med Oral Pathol Oral Radiol Endod* 1997;83:393–399.

Rao VM. Imaging of the temporomandibular joint. *Semin Ultrasound CT MR* 1995;16:513–526.

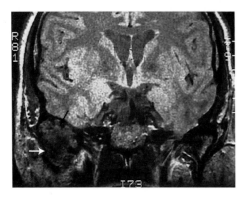

FIGURE 95.1A

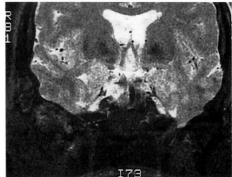

FIGURE 95.1B

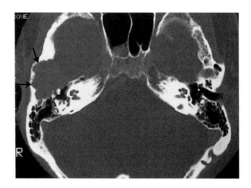

FIGURE 95.1C

CLINICAL HISTORY

A young adult patient presents with dizziness and hearing loss.

FINDINGS

Coronal proton density weighted images through the mandibular condyles show a destructive mass that is low in signal intensity. It appears to be eroding the adjacent temporal bone (Fig. 95.1A). On T2-weighted images, similar findings are present (Fig. 95.1B). The mass remains low in signal intensity. Axial CT images show the mass eroding the temporal bone and involving the anterior aspect of the epitympanum (Fig. 95.1C). (Images courtesy of Dr. Tim Larson.)

DIAGNOSIS

Central giant cell granuloma.

DISCUSSION

Giant cell granulomas are classified as central or peripheral according to location.

1. The central or intraosseous lesions are uncommon and controversy still exists regarding their pathophysiology. Some authors have proposed that these lesions be divided into aggressive and nonaggressive types (which has more clinical significance), rather than classifying them as two separate entities: giant cell granuloma (GCG) and giant cell tumor (GCT). Others think that GCG, GCT, and aneurysmal bone cyst represent a continuum of the same process, each lesion showing different degrees of aggressiveness modified by the age of the patient and location of the lesion. The term giant cell "reparative" granuloma, also once used to refer to this entity, has been discarded because the lesion does not appear to correspond to a reparative process.

2. The peripheral lesion, also called *epulis* (or fibroma), is more common and is seen in the soft tissues, usually the lingual or vestibular gingiva. Several repeated traumatic events have been proposed as predisposing factors, such as dental extraction and ill-fitting dentures. Imaging studies are usually not required in their evaluation or management.

Central giant cell granulomas are relatively rare lesions that may occur in the jaws or in the small bones of the hands and feet. In the jaw bones, they account for fewer than 7% of all benign lesions and they are more frequently seen in the mandible (two thirds of cases). The peak incidence is in the second and third decades. A female predominance is consistently reported.

The origin of giant cell granulomas is still the subject of speculation. The characteristic cell is the multinucleated giant cell, which some claim is derived from endothelial cell lines and others consider osteoclastic in origin. Favoring the later hypothesis is the fact that some GCG can be controlled using calcitonin therapy and that they share some similarity to brown tumors. Odontogenic origin has also been proposed because the lesion has a tendency to occur in dentulous areas at an age when there is an increased proliferation of these tissues. Nuclear inclusions seen on pathology suggest a viral etiology and are similar to those noted in Paget's disease. Trauma has never been proven to be a predisposing factor.

The hallmark of GCG is the presence of giant cells in an exuberant fibrous matrix. Brown tumor and cherubism, although histologically similar to GCG and GCT, can be distinguished clinically: Brown tumor has typical laboratory values and cherubism has a typical clinicoradiologic picture. Whenever a giant cell lesion is diagnosed on fine-needle aspiration, serum calcium and parathormone serum levels should be determined to rule out hyperparathyroidism.

Imaging is best performed with plain radiographs and CT. In the earlier stages, GCG can be unilocular with a well-defined sclerotic margin. As the lesion grows, it may become multilocular and expansile, showing progressively more aggressive features. As with other mandibular lesions, CT is used to evaluate the lesion's extent, integrity of the cortex, and the relationship to nearby teeth. Periosteal reaction may be seen, particularly when the cortex has been breached; soft tissue extension is also a possibility. The matrix of the tumor shows enhancement.

MRI may differentiate this lesion from aneurysmal bone cysts, which usually show typical fluid–fluid levels related to degradation of hemoglobin. Otherwise, this technique offers no advantage in the differential diagnosis, with the lesion being hypointense on both T1- and T2-weighted images.

Giant cell granulomas are managed surgically. Depending on the size and aggressiveness of the lesion, GCGs can be managed with simple curettage or radical resection, with or without bone grafting. These lesions are benign and do not tend to recur when completely excised. Medical therapy with calcitonin, which has an inhibitory effect on osteoclasts, can lead to remission of GCG.

SUGGESTED READINGS

Bodner L, Bar-Ziv J. Radiographic features of central giant cell granuloma of the jaws in children. *Pediatr Radiol* 1996;26:148–151.

Kaffe I, Ardekian L, Taicher S, et al. Radiologic features of central giant cell granuloma of the jaws. *Oral Surg Oral Med Oral Pathol Oral Radiol Endod* 1996;81:720–726.

Katz JO, Underhill TE. Multilocular radiolucencies. *Dental Clin North Am* 1994;38:63–81.

Kaw YT. Fine needle aspiration cytology of central giant cell granuloma of the jaw. A report of two cases. *Acta Cytol* 1994;38:475–478.

Whitaker SB, Bouquot JE. Estrogen and progesterone receptor status of central giant cell lesions of the jaws. *Oral Surg Oral Med Oral Pathol* 1994;77:641–644.

Whitaker SB, Singh BB. Intraoral giant cell lesions: the peripheral and central forms of these entities. *Practical Periodontics Aesthetic Dentistry* 1995;7:41–47.

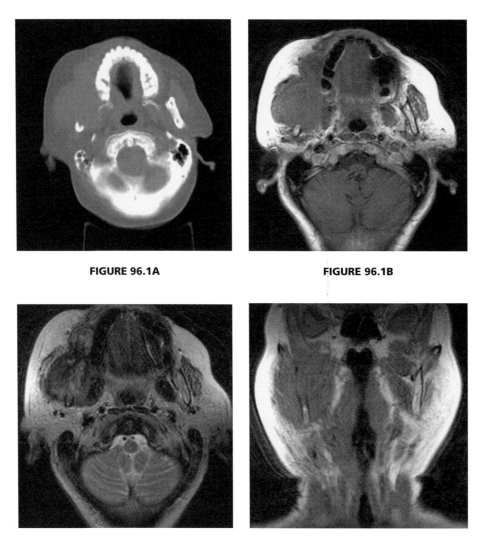

FIGURE 96.1A

FIGURE 96.1B

FIGURE 96.1C

FIGURE 96.1D

CLINICAL HISTORY

A 63-year-old man presents with pain, swelling, and numbness over the right jaw. Past medical history includes prior nephrectomy for renal cell carcinoma.

FINDINGS

Imaging of the mandible shows a destructive lesion of the masticator space involving the right ramus and mandibular angle (Fig. 96.1A–D). There is an associated soft tissue mass with replacement of the normal marrow signal seen on the coronal T1-weighted image.

DIAGNOSIS

Metastasis from renal cell carcinoma.

DISCUSSION

Metastasis to the mandible is rare, comprising less than 1% of all oral malignancies. Mandibular metastases can be the first sign of an occult malignancy (30% of cases), the first site of metastatic disease in a patient with a known primary (37%), or part of disseminated neoplasm. As in other bones, metastatic disease to the mandible is more prevalent between the fifth and seventh decades. The primary carcinomas that metastasize more frequently to the jaw mandible, in decreasing order of frequency, are breast, lung, kidney, thyroid, prostate, and gastric carcinomas. Mandibular involvement is 8 times more frequent than maxillar involvement, and the molar area is the most common site. Multifocality and bilaterality are rare.

Hematogenous dissemination results from impaction of embolized malignant cells in bone marrow vessels and depends on local vascular dynamics and marrow volume. According to several authors, inflammation may play a role in capturing blood-borne tumor cells, particularly to the apex of roots and dental sockets. The proliferating capillaries of granulation tissue have a fragmented basal membrane, which may be more permeable to tumor cells.

Frequent symptoms include pain, swelling, paresthesia, and loose teeth. On clinical examination, bony swelling with tenderness, teeth mobility, and trismus can be noted. Nonhealing of an extraction socket wound associated with a soft tissue mass extruding from the socket is another possible presentation and should be suspected in patients with known primary tumors. In the absence of prior history of cancer, benign considerations prevail, including fibroma, peripheral giant cell granuloma, and pyogenic granuloma.

The radiographic pattern depends on the primary tumor and can present as a lytic, blastic, or mixed lesion. The most frequent appearance is that of a solitary radiolucent lytic lesion with ill-defined margins. Purely blastic lesions are less frequent and more commonly seen in association with prostate cancer. The area of bone destruction can be localized or diffuse and show any pattern from a geographic lesion to a permeative process. Signs of aggressiveness include cortical disruption, periosteal reaction, associated soft tissue mass invading adjacent structures, and floating teeth (loss of lamina dura). Occasionally, a metastatic lesion of the mandible manifests as a pathologic fracture.

CT is optimal for demonstrating cortical disruption and loss of lamina dura but MRI is the most sensitive modality for detection of subtle bone marrow changes and invasion of soft tissues. Hypointensity of the bone marrow on T1-weighted images suggests bone marrow replacement and may be the first sign of metastatic bony involvement from hematogenous seeding. Invasion of the cortex is the first sign of involvement by direct extension and is well depicted on CT. Bone scintigraphy is used to detect and to determine the extent of metastatic bone disease.

Discovery of metastasis in the mandible is an ominous prognostic sign associated with a 30% 1-year survival rate. Nevertheless, early diagnosis allows appropriate therapy to be initiated. Therapy depends on the primary tumor site but typically consists of chemotherapy, radiotherapy, or hormonal therapy. Surgery is reserved for special cases in patients who are otherwise tumor free.

SUGGESTED READINGS

Johal AS, Davies SJ, Franklin CD. Condylar metastasis: a review and case report. *Br J Oral Maxillofac Surg* 1994;32:180–182.
Nortje CJ, van Rensburg LJ, Thompson IO. Case report. Magnetic resonance features of metastatic melanoma of the temporomandibular joint and mandible. *Dentomaxillofacial Radiol* 1996;25:292–297.

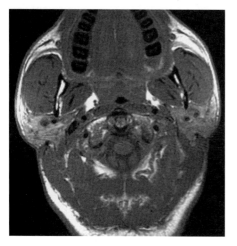

FIGURE 97.1A

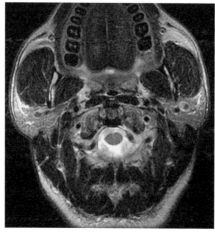

FIGURE 97.1B

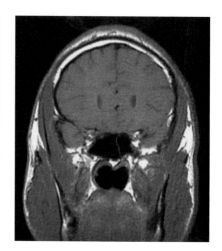

FIGURE 97.1C

CLINICAL HISTORY

A 25-year-old man presents with history of bilateral, painless cheek masses.

FINDINGS

Axial T1-weighted MRI of the midface shows diffuse, bilateral enlargement of the masseter muscles (Fig. 97.1A). The margins of the muscles are well defined and the signal characteristics are identical to the remainder of the other muscles on both T1- and T2-weighted images (Fig. 97.1B). No focal masses are noted. The parotid glands and Stenson's ducts are normal in appearance and no accessory parotid gland tissue is seen. The coronal view confirms these findings (Fig. 97.1C).

DIAGNOSIS

Benign masseteric hypertrophy.

DISCUSSION

Masseteric hypertrophy is an uncommon condition with an incidence twice as frequent in males as females. In more than half of cases, the condition is bilateral. A familial history may be present. Synonyms frequently used to refer to this condition include *idiopathic masseteric hypertrophy* and *masseteric pseudotumor*.

Patients usually present for cosmetic reasons with chronic, unilateral or bilateral cheek swelling. The condition is painless and does not compromise function. Clinical examination discloses unilateral or bilateral nontender masses in the buccomasseteric region, rubbery in consis-

tency, that become firm with teeth clenching. Accessory parotid gland tissue and prominent facial process of the parotid gland may be clinically indistinguishable from this condition, although they are usually softer in consistency and do not change consistency with contraction of the masseter muscles.

The pathophysiology of this condition is uncertain and both familial and acquired forms have been described. The acquired form is usually associated with some form of overuse of the masseter muscles such as chronic chewing, teeth clenching, bruxism (nocturnal teeth grinding), and malocclusion. Pathologically, the muscle shows an increase in size of the myocytes but is otherwise normal.

The role of imaging is to exclude pathologic processes that may present as a cheek mass and to evaluate for associated hypertrophy of other masticatory muscles. Ultrasound, CT, and MRI may be used.

CT better defines possible hypertrophy or exostoses of the mandibular angle at the site of insertion of the masseter muscle, which is a common associated finding, likely the result of overuse and overstimulation of this muscle. MRI, because of its better soft tissue resolution, is ideal for detecting any structural abnormalities or focal lesions within the muscle itself or in the surrounding structures.

Benign masseteric hypertrophy appears as diffuse enlargement of the masseter muscle with preservation of the muscle margins and no associated structural abnormalities. On MRI, the signal characteristics of the involved muscles are identical to those of the other muscles of mastication and no focal masses or areas of abnormal enhancement are seen. The pterygoid muscles may also be hypertrophied.

A potential imaging pitfall occurs when there is unilateral denervation atrophy of the masseter muscle and the contralateral muscle appears abnormally enlarged or masslike. This is usually due to an iatrogenic lesion of the masticator branch of V3 after surgery involving the bucco-masseteric region or due to perineural spread of a known malignancy.

Treatment of this condition is usually undertaken for cosmetic reasons. Conservative measures such as decreased stimulation of the masticatory muscles, including relaxation therapies and avoidance of chewing gums may be beneficial in some cases. Intramuscular injection of botulinic toxin have been attempted with variable success rates. Surgical treatment includes partial resection of the masseter muscles and mandibuloplasty via an extraoral or intraoral approach. The intraoral approach is preferred to avoid external scars and potential complications such as division of the marginal mandibular branch of the facial nerve and Stenson's duct. The most common complication of this surgery is transient postoperative trismus.

SUGGESTED READINGS

Honda T, Sasaki K, Takeuchi M, et al. Endoscope-assisted intraoral approach for masseteric hypertrophy. *Ann Plast Surg* 1997;38:9–14.

Mandel L, Kaynar A. Masseteric hypertrophy. *N Y S Dental J* 1994;60:44–47.

Moore AP, Wood GD. The medical management of masseteric hypertrophy with botulinum toxin type A. *Br J Oral Maxillofac Surg* 1994;32:26–28.

Morse MH. Enlargement of the pterygo-masseteric muscle complex. *Clin Radiol* 1994;49:71.

Nishida M, Iizuka T. Intraoral removal of the enlarged mandibular angle associated with masseteric hypertrophy. *J Oral Maxillofac Surg* 1995;53:1476–1479.

Rogers BA, Whear NM. Medical management of masseteric hypertrophy [letter; comment]. *J Oral Maxillofac Surg* 1995;53:492.

Rosa RA, Kotkin HC. That acquired masseteric look. *ASDC J Dentistry Child* 1996;63:105–107.

Smyth AG. Botulinum toxin treatment of bilateral masseteric hypertrophy. *Br J Oral Maxillofac Surg* 1994;32:29–33.

Tart RP, Kotzur IM, Mancuso AA, et al. CT and MR imaging of the buccal space and buccal space masses. *Radiographics* 1995;15:531–550.

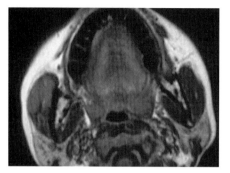

FIGURE 98.1A

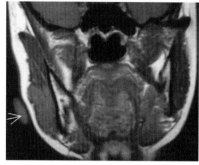

FIGURE 98.1B

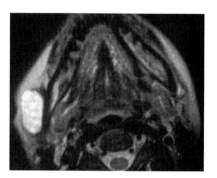

FIGURE 98.1C

CLINICAL HISTORY

A 38-year-old woman presents with a painless palpable mass on the right cheek.

FINDINGS

Axial and coronal T1-weighted (Fig. 98.1A, B) and axial fat-suppressed T2-weighted images show a mass within the right masseter muscle bulging the lateral contour of the muscle. The mass is lobulated in contour, does not remodel or erode the mandibular ramus, and does not extend into the buccal space. On T1-weighted images, it is slightly hyperintense to the remainder of the masseter muscle; on the T2-weighted image, it is very bright, showing some heterogeneity (Fig. 98.1C). Postgadolinium images (not shown) revealed intense enhancement.

DIAGNOSIS

Hemangioma of the right masseter muscle.

DISCUSSION

Hemangioma is the third most common cause of a buccomasseteric mass after normal variants of the parotid gland (facial processes and accessory parotid gland tissue) and masseteric hypertrophy. However, it is the most common benign tumor of this region, followed by lipoma and rhabdomyoma, and should be on the top of the list of differential diagnoses for a unilateral cheek mass.

Similar to hemangiomas in other locations, they may be of capillary, cavernous, mixed, or venous types. Whereas capillary hemangiomas are almost exclusively seen in children, cavernous and mixed types have a peak incidence between the third and fourth decades and have a slight female predominance.

Imaging is helpful both in the diagnosis and to evaluate the extent. On CT, hemangiomas present as well-defined masses that are hypodense to isodense to the masseter muscle and show intense contrast enhancement. Phleboliths may be present in the cavernous and venous varieties and are pathognomonic of this entity. MRI is the modality of choice to determine the full extent of the lesion. Clues to the diagnosis include the bright signal intensity on long repetition time (TR) images, the presence of serpentine flow voids within the lesion, and the intense gadolinium enhancement. Signal heterogeneity on T2-weighted images reflect the presence of fibrous and fatty septa interspersed between the vascular channels. Simple masseteric hemangioma should be distinguished from more complex hemangiomas, which may involve the buccomasseteric region and the masticator space and which show an intraosseous mandibular component, which have a different management and prognosis.

Because masseteric hemangiomas are benign, slow-growing tumors, they may remodel the adjacent bone or lead to reactive bony sclerosis, features not present in this case.

In this era of interventional radiology, most superficial facial hemangiomas are managed by in situ embolization using sclerosing agents, alone or preoperatively. Capillary type hemangiomas in a child are "leave me alone lesions" because they tend to regress spontaneously.

SUGGESTED READINGS

Boleo-Tome JP. Masseteric angioma. *Rev Port Estomatol Cir Maxilofac* 1966;7:81–87.

Cohen EK. MR imaging of soft tissue hemangiomas: correlation with pathologic findings. *Am J Radiol* 1988;150:1079–1081.

Klap P, Hadjean E, Negrier B, et al. Capillary-venous angioma of the temporo-masseteric region. *Ann Otolaryngol Chir Cervicofac* 1987;104:433–439.

Set PA, Somers JM, Britton PD, et al. Pictorial review: benign and malignant enlargement of the pterygo-masseteric muscle complex. *Clin Radiol* 1993;48:57–60.

Yonetsu K, Nakayama E, Yuasa K, et al. Imaging findings of some buccomasseteric masses. *Oral Surg Oral Med Oral Pathol Oral Radiol Endod* 1998;86:755–759.

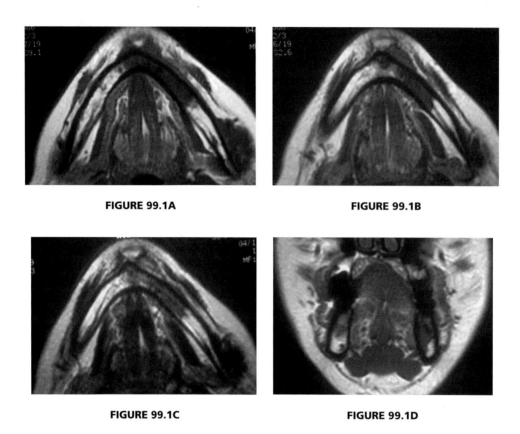

FIGURE 99.1A

FIGURE 99.1B

FIGURE 99.1C

FIGURE 99.1D

CLINICAL HISTORY

The patient is a 53-year-old woman complaining of numbness in the left side of the mandible and loose teeth.

FINDINGS

Axial T1-weighted (Fig. 99.1A, B) and T2-weighted images (Fig. 99.1C) and coronal T1-weighted images (Fig. 99.1D) show bone marrow infiltration of the mandibular symphysis and left parasymphyseal region and a small soft tissue mass in the vestibular space immediately to the left of the midline. The cortical bone is intact but abnormal soft tissue is shown within the inferior alveolar canal near the mental foramen, best shown on the coronal T1-weighted image. The mass is hypointense on both T1- and T2-weighted images, suggesting a highly cellular, or, alternatively, a highly fibrous tumor.

DIAGNOSIS

Mandibular lymphoma.

DISCUSSION

Primary lymphoma of bone is a rare entity, accounting for 5% of all extranodal lymphomas. In the head and neck region, extranodal lymphomas arise more commonly from the lymphoid tissue of the Waldeyer's ring, followed by the paranasal sinuses (PNS), orbits, oral cavity, and thyroid gland. Primary osseous lymphoma in the head and neck may arise from the mandible or maxilla, the premolar and molar regions of the mandible being reported as the most frequent sites. Pathologically, they are non-Hodgkin's lymphomas, usually of the large cell subtype. In the pediatric age group, Burkitt's lymphoma may also be seen in this region. The intraosseous tumor is thought to arise from remnants of lymphoid tissue that become entrapped during embryologic development.

Clinical findings are nonspecific and most often mimic inflammatory and infectious processes, as well as other neoplasms. Dental pain, mobile teeth, mandibular swelling, and facial numbness are the most frequent complaints. Therefore, most patients with this condition seek dental attention and not uncommonly are misdiagnosed with periapical diseases such as periodontitis. Dental radiographs and Panorex views of the mandible may show the "floating teeth" sign that results from resorption of the lamina dura and widening of the periodontal ligament space.

On cross-sectional imaging, findings are nonspecific, although there may be some clues to the diagnosis. MRI is the modality of choice to evaluate the extent of bone marrow replacement and to detect any associated soft tissue masses. Signal intensity is typical for a small cell, highly cellular tumor with poor water content, which translates as low signal intensity on long TR images. Perineural spread along the inferior alveolar nerve is not uncommon and serves as a conduit for tumor spread to the surrounding soft tissues.

However, biopsy is required to definitively differentiate other neoplasms including squamous cell carcinoma, malignancies of minor salivary gland origin, plasmacytoma, metastasis, and sarcomas. Imaging is also used to stage the disease. When the tumor is staged as IE (localized to a single extranodal site), such as in this case, the preferred treatment is radiation therapy or combined chemotherapy and radiation. The 5-year survival rate for extranodal non-Hodgkin's lymphoma of the maxillofacial region is 50% with a median expected survival of 10 years for patients with localized disease.

SUGGESTED READINGS

Barker GR. Unifocal lymphomas of the oral cavity. *Br J Maxillofac Surg* 1984;22:426–431.

Mincey DL. Primary malignant lymphoma of mandible: report of case. *J Oral Surg* 1974;32:221–224.

Robbins KT, Fuller LM, Manning J. Primary lymphoma of the mandible. *Head Neck Surg* 1986;8:192–196.

Ugar DA, Turker M, Memis L. Primary lymphoma of the mandible: report of a case. *J Maxillofac Surg* 1995;53:827–829.

Wolvius EB, Van der Valk P, Baart JA, et al. T-cell lymphoblastic lymphoma of the lower jaw in a young child. *Oral Surg Oral Med Oral Pathol* 1996;82:434–436.

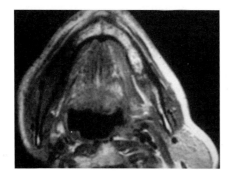

FIGURE 100.1A

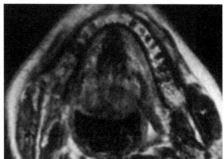

FIGURE 100.1B

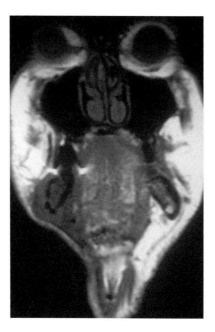

FIGURE 100.1C

CLINICAL HISTORY

A 72-year-old man with squamous cell carcinoma of the right external auditory canal, status post-surgery and radiation therapy, presents with a painful swelling of the right mandible.

FINDINGS

Axial T1- and T2-weighted and coronal T1-weighted images through the mandible (Fig. 100.1A–C) show bone marrow replacement of the right mandibular body, disruption of the outer cortex, and an associated soft tissue swelling. These changes extend from the parasymphyseal re-gion to the mandibular angle. In another patient, axial CT sections, soft tissue (Fig. 100.2A) and bone windows (Fig. 100.2B), show sclerosis and fragmentation of the left aspect of the mandibular body with cortical disruption of the outer and inner cortices and associated soft tissue edema.

DIAGNOSIS

Osteoradionecrosis of the mandible.

DISCUSSION

Osteoradionecrosis is a well-known sequela of radiation therapy. In order of decreasing frequency, the most affected sites in the head and neck region are the mandible, maxilla, and skull. The mandible is included in the radiation ports of several primary head and neck malignancies and nodal irradiation. Although the incidence of this grave sequela has significantly diminished because of improvements in radiation equipment and computerized radiation planning, it is still seen in 10% to 15% of patients receiving radiation therapy for head and neck neoplasms, more commonly for oral cavity tumors. The most common locations for osteoradionecrotic changes in the mandible are the molar and premolar areas and the retromolar buccal cortex.

This predisposition is related to blood supply, in that all these sites are dependent on the inferior alveolar artery and receive no collateral circulation because there are no muscular attachments.

The pathogenesis of this insult is primarily vascular. Radiation therapy produces hypovascular, hypoxic tissues, which are unable to compensate for tissue loss by means of intimal fibrosis and vascular thrombosis. There is also direct damage to the bone itself, particularly to the cellular elements with the higher metabolic rates (osteoblasts), leading to an imbalance between osteoblastic and osteoclastic activity. Radiation necrosis is a dose-dependent phenomenon. A dose of 60 Gray is considered the threshold above which radiation necrosis can occur independently of the presence of other predisposing factors. These include advanced age, atherosclerotic disease, poor dental hygiene, alcohol and tobacco use, and surgical or nonsurgical trauma, prior or soon after, radiation therapy. Sixty to eighty percent of cases follow dental extractions. Factors related to the therapy itself include high radiation dose, large radiation fields, and poor fractionation.

Pain, trismus, numbness, and difficulty chewing are the most frequent complaints. Soft tissue swelling is frequent when there is secondary infection or pathologic fracture. On clinical examination, the hallmark of osteoradionecrosis is the presence of exposed bone. Orocutaneous fistulas are commonly seen. Latency periods are variable and range from 3 months to as long as 20 years after radiotherapy.

Although plain films and CT are the preferred imaging modalities for diagnosis of radiation necrosis, MRI and bone scans are more sensitive because they may detect bone marrow changes and assess vascularity. On MRI, bone marrow edema and replacement by necrotic tissue manifests as loss of the T1-weighted hyperintensity of fatty marrow and an increase in the T2-weighted signal. There may be associated cortical disruption and pathologic fracture. MRI is also the best modality for detecting any associated soft tissue changes. In the early stages, CT may show bony sclerosis and periosteal thickening. As the disease progresses, a mixed radiolucent-sclerotic pattern ensues, followed by diffuse rarefaction with cortical disruption and bone fragmentation. Enhancing soft tissue may be seen adjacent to pathologic fractures and can be mistaken by recurrent tumor. However, discrepancy between the size of the soft tissue mass and the site of bony destruction favors radiation necrosis. Gas bubbles, once thought to be pathognomonic of secondary infection, can be seen in osteoradionecrosis associated with dehiscence of the overlying mucosa, with air tracking into the bony defect. Cortical disruption is more commonly seen in the buccal cortex in patients who undergo treatment with external beam radiation.

Differential diagnosis of an irregular mixed mandibular lesion includes primary and secondary malignancies, osteomyelitis, and radiation necrosis. In this particular clinical setting (prior radiation to the neck), the major challenge is to differentiate tumor recurrence from radiation necrosis. This may be impossible upon the basis of clinical and radiologic assessment alone and fine-needle aspiration is often required.

Management of radiation necrosis depends on the extent of bony necrosis and usually requires debridement of necrotic bone and reconstruction with myocutaneous flaps or bone grafts.

SUGGESTED READINGS

Bachmann G, Rossler R, Klett R, et al. The role of magnetic resonance imaging and scintigraphy in the diagnosis of pathologic changes in the mandible after radiation therapy. *Int J Oral Maxillofac Surg* 1996;25:189–195.

Carlson ER. The radiobiology, treatment and prevention of osteoradionecrosis of the mandible. *Rec Res Cancer Res* 1994;134:191–199.

Curi MM, Dib LL. Osteoradionecrosis of the jaws: a retrospective study of the background factors and treatment in 104 cases. *J Oral Maxillofac Surg* 1997;55:540 544.

Hermans R, Fossion E, Ioannides C, et al. CT findings in osteoradionecrosis of the mandible. *Skeletal Radiol* 1996;25:31–36.

Rabin BM, Meyer JR, Berlin JW, et al. Radiation-induced changes in the central nervous system and head and neck. *Radiographics* 1996;16:1055–1072.

SUBJECT INDEX

Cavernous hemangioma, of left orbit
(contd.)
treatment of, 117
vision loss with, 116–117, 116f
treatment of, 107
Cavernous sinus, intraorbital meningioma
with extension to, 108–109, 108f.
See also Intraorbital meningioma
Central nervous system (CNS), lesions of, in
neurofibromatosis I, 119
Cephalocele(s)
basal, 41
described, 41
occipital, 41
sincipital, 41
trans-sphenoidal, 40–41, 40f. See also
Trans-sphenoidal cephalocele
Cepholomeningocele(s), described, 41
Cheek mass, painless
with accessory parotid gland, 152–153,
152f
and benign masseteric hypertrophy,
226–227, 226f
with pleomorphic adenoma, 140–141,
140f
Cheek swelling, and malignant otitis
externa, 190–192, 190f
Chemodectoma(s), 65. See also Glomus
tumors
Children
congenital laryngeal cysts in, 32–33
optic nerve glioma in, 115
primary tracheal tumors in, 75
Cholesteatoma(s), developmental, 212–213,
212f. See also Epidermoid(s)
Cholesterol cyst. See Cholesterol granuloma
Cholesterol granuloma, 208–209, 208f
described, 209
differential diagnosis of, 209
hemorrhage with, 209
histopathologic examination of, 209
lateral gaze diplopia with, 208–209, 208f
pathogenesis of, 209
source of, 209
Chordoma, clival. See Clival chordoma
Choroidal (uveal) melanoma, 98–99, 98f
causes of, 99
treatment of, 99
vision loss with, 98–99, 98f
Clival chordoma, 2f–3f, 3–4
composition of, 4
described, 3
histology of, 3–4
MRI signal characteristics of, 4
presenting symptoms of, 3
radiologic evaluation of, 4
sites of, 3
treatment of, 4
CNS. See Central nervous system (CNS)
Computed tomography (CT). See specific
disorders
Congenital laryngeal cysts, in children,
32–33
Cough, chronic
with primary tracheal squamous
carcinoma, 74–75, 74f
and vallecular cyst, 18–19, 18f

Cranial nerve paralysis, and paraganglioma,
200–201, 200f
Craniovertebral junction metastasis, 6–7, 6f
categories of, 7
CT with MRI in, 7
features of, 7
management of, 7
setting of, 7
CT. See Computed tomography (CT)
Cyst(s)
bone, aneurysmal, 12–13, 12f–13f. See
also Aneurysmal bone cyst (ABC)
branchial cleft, second, 56–58, 56f, 57f,
96–97, 96
cholesterol. See Cholesterol granuloma
dermoid, described, 133
epidermoid, of floor of mouth, 132–133,
132f
lymphoepithelial, benign, HIV-
associated, 142–143, 142f. See
also Benign lymphoepithelial cysts
(BLCs), HIV-associated
retention, vs. mucoceles, 179
saccular, vs. laryngocele, 29
thyroglossal duct, 68–69, 68f, 86–87,
86f. See also Thyroglossal duct
cyst
tornwaldt, 34–35, 34f. See also Tornwaldt
cyst
vallecular, 18–19, 18f. See also Vallecular
cyst

D

Deafness, glomus jugulare tumor and,
216–217, 216f
Dermoid cysts. See also Epidermoid cyst
described, 133
Diplopia, lateral gaze, with cholesterol
granuloma, 208–209, 208f
Dizziness
and central giant cell carcinomas,
222–223, 222f
with trans-sphenoidal cephalocele, 40–41,
40f
Dysphagia
with pyriform sinus carcinoma, 26–27,
26f
and squamous cell carcinoma of base of
left tongue, 124–126, 124f
in vagus nerve schwanoma in post-styloid
compartment of parapharyngeal
space, 78–79, 78f
Dyspnea, with bilateral fluid-filled
laryngoceles, 32–33

E

Epidermoid(s), 212–213, 212f
clinical presentation of, 213
composition of, 213
differential diagnosis of, 213
prevalence of, 213
sites of, 213
source of, 213
trigeminal nerve paresthesia and,
212–213, 212f
Epidermoid cyst, of floor of mouth,
132–133, 132f

Epistaxis, and esthesioneuroblastoma,
182–184, 182f
Epstein-Barr virus, antibodies against, and
squamous cell carcinoma of
nasopharynx, 43
Epulis, 223
Esthesioneuroblastoma(s), 182–184, 182f
age as factor in, 183
bimodal distribution of, 183
described, 183
differential diagnosis of, 183–184
epistaxis with, 182–184, 182f
nasal obstruction with, 182–184, 182f
treatment of, 184
Exophthalmus, painless, bilateral,
progressive, in thyroid
orbitopathy, 110–111, 110f
Ex-pleomorphic adenoma, 140–141

F

Facial fullness, painless, and Warthin's
tumor of parotid gland, 154–155,
154f
Facial mass, with high-grade
mucoepidermoid carcinoma of
parotid gland, 156–157, 156f
Facial nerve, weakness of, in adenoid cystic
carcinoma of parotid gland with
perineural extension along facial
nerve into temporal bone,
144–145, 144f
Facial nerve palsy
and facial nerve schwannoma, 194–195,
194f
with Ramsay-Hunt syndrome, 196–197,
196f
Facial nerve schwannoma, 194–195, 194f
clinical findings with, 195
described, 194
facial nerve palsy with, 194–195, 194f
incidence of, 194
manifestations of, 195
treatment of, 195
twitching with, 194–195, 194f
Facial pain
left-sided, and trigeminal schwannoma,
16–17, 16f
and petroclival meningioma, 8
and trigeminal nerve schwannoma, 10
Facial paresthesias
left-sided, and trigeminal schwannoma,
16–17, 16f
and petroclival meningioma, 8
and trigeminal nerve schwannoma, 10
Facial process of the parotid gland, 162
Fibrovascular polyp
described, 136
of oropharynx, 136–137, 136f. See also
Oropharynx, fibrovascular polyp
of
Floor of mouth
epidermoid cyst of, 132–133, 132f
site of, 133
swelling of, 132–133, 132f
in lingual thyroid, 130–131, 130f
with sialolithiasis of left submandibular
gland, 158–159, 158f
Frey syndrome, 139

Tracheal squamous carcinoma, primary, 74–75, 74f
  in children, 75
Tracheal tumors, clinical manifestations of, 74–75, 74f
Transglottic carcinoma, defined, 25
Transglottic squamous cell carcinoma, of larynx, 24–25, 24f
Trans-sphenoidal cephalocele, 40–41, 40f
  age as factor in, 41
  classification of, 41
  dizziness with, 40–41, 40f
  headaches with, 40–41, 40f
  treatment of, 41
Trauma
  and aneurysmal bone cyst, 13
  larngeal, findings in, 30–31
Trigeminal nerve paresthesia, and epidermoids, 212–213, 212f
Trigeminal nerve schwannoma, 10–11, 10f, 16–17, 16f
  composition of, 11
  described, 17
  differential diagnosis of, 17
  facial pain and, 10, 16–17, 16f
  facial paresthesias and, 10, 16–17, 16f
  management of, 11, 17
  and neurofibromatosis type II, 16–17
  presentation of, 11
  sites of, 11
  size of, 17
Trismus, and malignant otitis externa, 190–192, 190f
Tumor(s). *See also specific types*
  laryngeal, classification of, 25
  tracheal, clinical manifestations of, 74–75, 74f
  Warthin's, of parotid gland, 154–155, 154f
Twitching, and facial nerve schwannoma, 194–195, 194f
Tympanogenic infections, and labyrinthitis, 215

U

Unilateral buccomasseteric masses
  bilateral accessory parotid glands and, 162
  differential diagnosis of, 163
Uveal melanoma, 98–99, 98f

V

Vagus nerve schwannoma
  in post-styloid compartment of parapharyngeal space, 78–79, 78f
    differential diagnosis of, 79
    pathology of, 78–79
    symptoms of, 78
    treatment of, 79
  prevalence of, 78
Vallecular cyst, 18–19, 18f
  in adults, 19
  cough and, 18–19, 18f
  described, 19
  differential diagnosis of, 19
  in infants, 19
  laryngomalacia and, 19
  management of, 19
Vestibular schwannoma, 204–205, 204f
  bilatera, and neurofibromatosis type II, 188–189, 188f
  described, 205
  differential diagnosis of, 205
  hearing loss with, 204–205, 204f
  intracanalicular, 198–199, 198f. *See also* Intracanalicular vestibular schwannoma
  management of, 205
  prevalence of, 205
  sites of, 199
  symptons of, 205
  tinnitus with, 204–205, 204f
Vision loss
  with cavernous hemangioma of left orbit, 116–117, 116f
  with choroidal melanoma, 98–99, 98f
  with intraorbital meningioma with extension to cavernous sinus, 108–109, 108f

with optic nerve glioma, 114–115, 114f
  progressive, with neurofibromatosis type II, 206–207, 206f
Visual acuity, decreased, with radiation-induced optic neuropathy, 12–113, 112f
Vocal cord, squamous cell carcinoma of, 20–21, 20f
  causes of, 21
  nodal spread with, 21
  treatment of, 21
  types of, 21
Vocal cord paralysis, 22–23, 22f
  causes of, 23
  recurrent laryngeal nerve in, 23
  right, Riedel's thyroiditis with, 88–90, 88f
Voice, weakness in, and chronic posttraumatic deformity of larynx, 30–31, 30f

W

Warthin's tumor
  of parotid gland, 154–155, 154f
    composition of, 155
    cystic changes in, 155
    facial fullness and, 154–155, 154f
    lymph node involvement in, 155
    prevalence of, 155
    site of, 155
    treatment of, 155
Wegener's granulomatosis, and nasal lymphoma, 166

X

Xerostomia, in Sjögren's syndrome, 150–151, 150f

Z

Zimmermann, pericytes of, hemangiopericytomas from, 177